Moms with ADD

Moms with ADD
A Self-Help Manual

Christine A. Adamec

Foreword by Esther Gwinnell, M.D.

TAYLOR TRADE PUBLISHING

Lanham • New York • Oxford

Designed by Janis Owens

TAYLOR TRADE PUBLISHING
An Imprint of the Rowman & Littlefield Publishing Group
4501 Forbes Boulevard, Suite 200
Lanham, MD 20706

Distributed by National Book Network

The material in *Moms with ADD* is nor intended to be, nor should it be construed as, medical advice. Consult your physician or therapist for information on attention deficit disorders.

Library of Congress Cataloging-in-Publication Data

Adamec, Christine A., 1949–
  Moms with ADD/by Christine Adamec.
   p. cm.
  Includes bibliographical references.
  ISBN 0-87833-175-1 (pbk.)
  1. Attention-deficit disorder in adults. 2. Mothers—Mental health. 3. Attention-deficit disordered adults—Family relationships. I. Title.

RC394.A85 A33 2000
616.85'89—dc21   00-044684

Printed in the United States of America

Acknowledgments

Thanks first to my husband, John Adamec, for constantly boosting my morale and supporting this project. I am also grateful to the following people, who provided invaluable assistance: Terry Matlen, M.S.W., of Ann Arbor, Michigan—ADD coach, therapist, and creative, helpful person; Jerri Jenista, M.D.—pediatrician and mother of five from Ann Arbor, Michigan; Kathleen Nadeau, Ph.D.—psychologist, author, and co-editor of *ADDvance*, a wonderful magazine for women with ADD; Sari Solden—therapist, author, and pioneer in recognizing women with ADD, and Kate Kelly—author and ADD coach with many innovative ideas.

Special thanks to my editor, Camille Cline, for her excellent editing of the manuscript and her sensitivity to the issues that moms with ADD face.

Christine Adamec

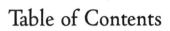

Table of Contents

Foreword   xiii

Part One

ADD Moms in a Non-ADD World:
Practical Coping Strategies   1

1 The Key to ADD: Basic Issues   3
   Still a New Concept: Girls and Women Can Have ADD
   It's Hard to Be a Mom with ADD
   Some People Still Think ADD Is a Myth
   What the World Expects from All Mothers
   Moms with ADD: What the World Usually Gets
   How Experts Diagnose ADD
   Sari Solden Screening Checklist for Women with ADD

2 Zeroing in on the Good Aspects of ADD   19
   Hyperfocusing
   Curiosity
   Creativity and Spontaneity: Nonlinear Thinking
   Compassion, Sensitivity, and Empathy
   Sense of Humor
   High Energy: When the Energizer Mom Keeps Going and Going
   Living in the Now
   Deep Commitment to Children
   Multitasking Ability

3 Working on Solutions to Common ADD Problems   31
Lost in Space: Organizational Problems and Solutions
Why Am I Always Losing Things?
Saying Yes Too Much
Time: It Isn't That Flexible Except on Star Trek
Mom, Are You Zoning Out Again? Learning to Listen
Blurting Out Comments: Getting a Grip on that Tongue
Hyperreactivity to Stimuli
High- and Low-Tech Solutions Can Help

4 Juggling Family and Work: The Family   57
Analyzing Donna
Create a Plan
Skills to Work on at Home
Be Firm: Sometimes Moms with ADD "Wimp Out"
Working Out Solutions with Family Members
Don't Forget Boundaries! Yours and Theirs

5 Juggling Family and Work: The Workplace   69
Finding and Evaluating Childcare
Is Your Job ADD-Unfriendly?
Work Is Still There When You're at Home
Laws That Affect Workers Today

Part Two

Family Matters   77

6 Your Children Have ADD—Or Don't   79
Your Children Have ADD Too
Your Children Don't Have ADD
Some of Your Children Have ADD—And Some Don't

7 You Have A Baby: But What If You Have ADD Too?   93
Babies/Toddlers
Limits—with Love
Your Own Expectations as a New Mom

8 Parenting The School-Age Child: The Basics   103
Realities of Parenting
Organizational Nightmares

It's a Two-Way Interaction: Children Affect Parents Too
Create Rules and Stick with Them

9 The ADD Mom and The Adolescent: Now *There* Is a Challenge! 115
Adolescent Angst vs. Plain-Old Bad Behavior
Considering Boundaries and Expectations
Adapting to Your Teenager's Changing Needs
Disciplining Your Adolesent: Choices Are Important

10 School Daze: Your Child Goes to School 123
Helping Your Child Adjust
If Problems Arise
Parent-Teacher Conferences
Homework Headaches and Science Project Nightmares
When the System Is Not the Solution: Charter Schools
Home Schooling
If Your Child Has ADD: School Requirements
If the School Absolutely Refuses to Cooperate: What One
   Parent Tried that Worked

Part Three

Special Struggles 143

11 Coping With Difficult or Painful Emotions that May Accompany ADD 145
Anger: Your Temper and Your Child's Misbehavior
Self-Blame and Guilt
Frustration and Feelings of Incompetence
Stress
Fears of ADD Making You a Bad Mother
Traits of Bad Mothers
Could It Be Something Else?

12 Coping With Holidays and Other Tough Times 159
The Holidays
Children's Birthdays or Special Parties
Summer Vacations from School

Travel Joys and Woes
When Your Children Are Sick

Part Four

Getting Outside Help   165

13 Professional Help   167
Self-Test: Should You Consider Seeking Therapy?
Medical Doctors: From General Practitoners to Psychiatrists
Psychologists: What They Can and Cannot Do
What If the "Expert" Says You Don't Have ADD?
Finding a Good Professional

14 Medications That May Help   175
Fear of Taking "Drugs"
ADD-Specific Medications
Other Medications
How Doctors Select Medications for ADD
Pros and Cons of Medication
How Do You Know If the Medicine Is Working?
"Natural" or Alternative Medicines
Dietary Changes
Homeopathy and Biofeedback

15 Support Groups, Coaching and Other
Forms of Help for the Mom with ADD   187
Professional organizers
ADD Coaches
Support Groups: What They Are and Can Do

Appendix A: Recommended Books   191

Appendix B: Magazines and Journals   193

Appendix C: National Organizations   195

Appendix D: Support Groups for Adults with ADD   197

Appendix E: Websites and Listservs   201

Appendix F: Summer Camps with Programs for Kids with ADD   203

Appendix G: State Contacts for Charter
School Information   205

Appendix H: Products That May Be Helpful   209

Bibliography   211

Index   217

Foreword

Once upon a time, doctors believed that attention deficit/hyperactivity disorder (ADHD) was a disease of childhood. At the age of 18, children who had been hyperactive were supposed to magically heal or be cured and not require medication or treatment any more. This is what I was taught in medical school, and as is often the way with fairy tales, I learned later that this happy ending was not true.

I was also taught in medical school that girls rarely experienced ADHD, and that this diagnosis was overwhelmingly found among preadolescent boys. No one mentioned that adult women could have ADHD—such a diagnosis just did not occur to anyone. We now know that girls can and do have ADHD. We also know that when these girls grow up, the ADHD does not magically vanish, and many still struggle. Many adult women with ADHD have children with attention deficits as well.

I served six years as medical director for Project Network, a residential drug and alcohol treatment program for pregnant addicts. Our treatment program—in an old converted apartment building—included not only the mothers but also all their children under the age of six. I coordinated psychiatric and medical treatment for the mothers and their children, and supervised the child treatment program staff. It gave me a whole new appreciation for the word *chaos*.

Of course, the children in this program had more than attention deficit disorder (ADD) to deal with. They had usually been in foster care at least one time, their mothers were addicted to drugs and alcohol, and more than half of the children had been exposed to street drugs before they were born. The ADHD was just one more problem they had to find a way to cope with.

Not only did the children have ADHD, more than a third of their mothers had it, too. Some of the methamphetamine addicts were clearly "self-treating" their problems of attention, impulsivity, and disorganization with stimulants. The street drugs the mothers were taking were sometimes necessary for them to function in very ordinary ways. For example, these mothers came to us without knowing how to clean house, or how to keep track of important papers. They had trouble controlling their impulses, and would blurt out comments in the riskiest situations.

One woman was so impulsive in her behavior that she could not prevent herself from making comments on other women's clothing or hairstyles—no matter how insulting the comment might sound. She was in the program only three days before she got smacked in the face by another client.

We started out thinking we would do drug treatment, but quickly found that we had to teach our women most of the things Christine Adamec covers in *Moms with ADD*. We had coaches to help with learning how to get organized; how to clean house; and how to fill out and keep track of welfare forms, bus tickets, and meeting slips. We developed parenting classes and helped mothers with ADD learn to manage their hyperactive children. I wish this book had been available then.

Over the years I have found more adults in my general psychiatric practice who have ADD or ADHD. The magic didn't work for them, I guess. Their adult lives were plagued with mildewed laundry because "mom got distracted." One patient had lost five jobs in four years for lateness, procrastination, losing important papers, or being disorganized in general. Her desk looked like a paper bomb had gone off—but her brilliance in computer program design kept getting her a new job. She was smart, but her ADD was destroying her life.

If you add a child or two, or possibly a *hyperactive* child or two, to the mixture, ADHD can become an even greater burden. And since, as Ms. Adamec points out, ADHD tends to run in families, the odds are good that if you have ADHD, so will one or more of your children.

Medications have helped enormously, and the slow trend toward accepting that adults might still *need* medication has benefited thousands. But the medication is far from perfect. Some people can't tolerate the medicine, and most people get only a partial response. Even with good response to, say, Dexedrine, my patients still have trouble finding their car keys or remembering appointments. Even remembering to take their medication is a problem. So as with most medical problems that medical science can't cure, people have to find ways to cope.

I regularly recommend self-help books for my patients. I look for books that are practical, optimistic, and designed for the needs of the people who read them. *Moms with ADD* is *designed* to be useful to women with ADD who are struggling with the stereotype of the perfect mother. I think it will also be useful for fathers with ADD, or cousins with ADD. It's pretty hard for my ADHD patients to read a book from cover to cover. Ms. Adamec has created a book that can be dipped into, used as a reference text, or serve as a kind of "cookbook" for coping.

If you have problems with housework, there's a clearly written section on just getting organized. If you blurt out unpleasant "truths," Chapter Two has practical suggestions for managing that. If you have lost the last 37 permission slips for your child's field trips, Ms. Adamec makes it possible to easily find them and get advice for doing it differently next time. If you feel chronically guilty because you just can't live up to that perfect mother celebrated on stage and screen, you will find comfort and empathy in every chapter.

More than just practical advice, this book also brings out the positive aspects of

ADD. The creativity of my ADHD patients, their ability to live in the moment, and the way they think "outside the box" have given their families great joy. I am always glad when I see that the treatment has not squelched that. I'm glad to see that this book remembers and revels in those special qualities.

There is no requirement that you read this book from cover to cover, in order. Read what's important *right now,* and you will get an education about ADHD that will help you. You can start with Chapter Four about Juggling Family and Work, browse the extensive resource list at the end of the book, and then go back to Chapter Nine about The ADD Mom and the Adolescent. With this education about ADD under your belt, you should be able to navigate the wilderness of doctors, teachers, and babysitters that you must deal with every day.

And finally, *Moms with ADD* has enough important information for coping with the chaos of family life that it can be useful to moms *without* ADD. If you have young children, a job, daycare and only two hands, this book has some pragmatic approaches to parenting that can benefit *any* mom.

Esther Gwinnell, M.D.

ADD Moms in a Non-ADD World

Practical Coping Strategies

Part One defines key problems faced by moms with ADD and offers practical coping solutions. It also includes information on some good (yes, there are some!) aspects of attention deficit disorder, which when mobilized can bring positive results.

The Key to ADD: Basic Issues

Just about *everyone* knows that only boys have attention deficit disorder (ADD)—because girls are always nice and neat and, of course, very organized. And of course *everybody* knows that although some of these boys will grow up to be men with ADD—those nice, neat, and organized girls will grow up to become women who have it all together as well-organized adults.

Except for one problem: Everybody who believes my first paragraph is wrong. Many girls can and do have ADD, and they grow up to be women who are not at all neat and organized. They may instead be quite messy people, albeit intensely creative individuals.

▶ STILL A NEW CONCEPT: GIRLS AND WOMEN CAN HAVE ADD

Only in the past few years has there been any true acknowledgment that girls and woman can experience ADD, starting with the groundbreaking book *Women with Attention Deficit Disorder* by therapist and fellow ADDer Sari Solden. One reason why people didn't know about girls and women with ADD is that nearly all research was done on boys and men with ADD. In a self-fulfilling prophecy, researchers studied only the people who they *knew* were the primary group with ADD (boys and men) and thus continued to perpetuate the myth that ADD was exclusively a male issue.

Researchers have finally begun to realize that many girls and women also struggle with ADD. It may be noticed less because many are "inattentive," rather than hyperactive. They aren't bouncing off walls and aggravating everyone. Instead, girls and women with ADD may be quietly inattentive, doing what my son calls "zoning out."

In some cases, girls are hyperactive. As children, they're seen as "tomboys," and as women, they're perceived as highly energetic or manic. They may have ADD instead.

▶ IT'S HARD TO BE A MOM WITH ADD

It's also true that women with ADD share traits that can sometimes make it hard to function optimally, especially when you also hold the role of mother. Traits such as distractibility, disorganization, impulsivity, and the already-mentioned inattentiveness don't seem useful when you are trying to rear one or more children in our non-ADD world. In this world, you're supposed to color inside the lines, go slow, and eat all your vegetables—among various other expected standard behaviors.

It's hard to be someone seen mostly as a person who forgets everything, is off on her own planet, or is foolishly impulsive and sometimes just plain silly. The name-calling can be tough: ditsy, absent-minded, space cadet, or worse—crazy or lazy. I know this intellectually and I also know it personally, as do most of my readers.

A former classmate told me, "We knew you didn't take drugs back in college. But we figured that you didn't need them! You were already 'there' all by yourself." She was talking about a hallmark of many with attention deficit disorder—the inattentive driftiness. Ironically, taking "drugs" can often make us well aware and attentive.

Moms Usually Get Blamed When Problems Occur

Another reason it's hard to be a mother with ADD is that in today's society, it's hard to be a mother, period. Read or watch nearly any story about children with problems, and you can rely on the ensuing speculation or outright statements that the underlying problem is really bad parents. Which means, to most people, bad mothers. She was too aggressive. Or too weak. Or overly involved. Or not involved enough. Someone recently told me about a refrigerator magnet that said, "If it's not bacterial or viral, it's maternal." Meaning, it's nearly always mom's fault.

It's mom's fault if the child goes to school and gets sick: She should have noticed that he wasn't feeling well. It's mom's fault if her daughter is having trouble with some of her classes or arguing with friends.

Since most mothers get blamed for problems with children, what about mothers with attention deficit disorder? I think you can guess: They often make easy and obvious targets for heavy-duty blame. If a non-ADD mother is presumed guilty for all childhood trials and tribulations, how much guiltier is the ADD mother? A lot more.

And if the child has ADD, the blame is even more likely to be extended. Yet the only valid "blame" is usually a genetic one, although we can hardly be rationally faulted for our genes.

Moms and Guilt: How Society Sees Them

Situation	Judgment of Mom
Your child is late for school.	Mothers should make sure their children are on time. Mom is guilty.
Your child is kind to another.	The child is nice. Or gesture is not seen. Credit to Mom: 0
Your 4-year-old has a tantrum in the supermarket.	Why can't mothers today control their kids? Mom is guilty.
Child receives an A on report.	Child is smart and hard-working. Credit to Mom: 0
Child receives an F on report.	Mother probably doesn't care enough to help child. Maybe she has other problems too. Mom is guilty.

Charts, Graphs, and Complicated Parenting: Too Tough for the Mom with ADD

Another reason why parenting can be difficult for the ADD mom lies within the plethora of confusing and conflicting advice mothers are given. For example, if you read parenting books, most of them recommend strategies and exercises that can be impossible for the mother with ADD. And if you have a child with ADD and read some of those parenting books, watch out! The complex charts and elaborate point systems that such books recommend make most mothers with ADD throw up their hands.

There is no perfect parenting model for the mother with attention deficit disorder to follow. But there are methods that work, and it is possible to adapt recommendations of experts. For example, most parenting books advise that your child should have a quiet place to do homework. He should sit there and work straight through until done. He should not have his TV and radio blaring.

Yet sometimes that kind of noise and those frequent breaks work extremely well for the child with ADD, just as sometimes they work for the mom with ADD. We need to rethink what works and what doesn't—both for us as parents and for our children too.

▶ SOME PEOPLE STILL THINK ADD IS A MYTH

Another blot on our horizon is that there are still people who think attention deficit disorder is a myth, and that boys and girls who are very active or dreamy are just normal kids. Or they are messed up because they have such dysfunctional and terrible mothers. Such people equate ADD as a "disease of the month" or trendy fad.

Do I Have ADD?

Many people also think, hey, sometimes *I* forget my keys or *I* am late for an appointment or *I* act impulsively—and that is true. Most people display such behavior occasionally. But not to an extent that they face constant, serious disruptions to their lives. To explain further, I've created a simple chart.

ADD-Like Behaviors in Average People vs. People with ADD

Behavior	Average person	Person with ADD*
Loses keys (they're gone)	Once a year, at most	Four or five times a year
Forgets important appointments	Two to three times a year	At least monthly
Blurts out remarks that distress others	Once a month at most	At least weekly
Constantly moving about; can't sit still	Not a problem	If person with ADD is hyperactive, a problem much of the time
Periods of attentiveness	An hour or two	A few minutes or, if very interested in task, 3–4 hours
Can think of creative ideas	Several a week	Constantly has ideas; it's sorting them out that is the problem
Late for work or other appointment	Rarely	Frequently
Agrees to do three things in same timeframe	Rarely	Frequently. Tries to do them all. Sometimes succeeds!
Loses important papers like checks	Rarely	Up to once a month

*Person with ADD who has not developed accommodations to solve problems and/or is not taking ADD medications.

It Takes Time for Acceptance to Come

It wasn't long ago that many people believed clinical depression was an excuse for people to get out of work or make people feel sorry for them. Other people equated depression with a really bad mood. It's true everyone feels "down" sometimes, but major depression is far more magnified and permanent than a sad mood that passes.

Only recently has the public begun to realize depression is a real illness with effective treatments. Eventually, the naysayers will realize the same kind of truths hold for ADD. It's real and it's more than a passing problem. There are medications and strategies that help people with ADD, just as there are treatments for depression.

Another problem with gaining acceptance of ADD is that you can't get a blood or urine test for it. No lab tests definitively say, "Yes! She has ADD!" But scientists have noted distinct brain differences in the dopamine levels of adults with and without ADD, and as recently as 1999, findings have been published in such prestigious medical journals as the *Lancet*.

But it's too expensive for everyone who might have ADD to get a special brain test. Until better diagnostic tools are developed, we must rely on psychologists and psychiatrists who can recognize ADD—just as we rely on doctors to diagnose depression and other problems that are accepted but can't be diagnosed with a blood or urine test.

HOW MANY MOMS HAVE ATTENTION DEFICIT DISORDER?

No one knows for sure how many mothers have attention deficit disorder. However, we can make educated guesses. For example, if we conservatively assume that at least five million children in the United States have ADD, an extrapolation can be made.

Recent unpublished research by Craig W. Walker, Ph.D., a Montana clinical psychologist on the ADHD Gender Study Project, found a genetic component in about half the biological parent pairs of children he studied. Dr. Walker told me that he found that when a parent has ADHD, it is about equally likely to be the biological mother or father. This means about 25 percent of the children have mothers with ADHD and about 25 percent have fathers with ADHD.

Generalizing this number to the large population of children with ADHD, there are about 1,250,000 mothers with ADHD in the United States (25 percent of five million children). For further information, contact Dr. Walker at his e-mail address: veloce@digisys.net.

▶ WHAT THE WORLD EXPECTS FROM ALL MOTHERS

Here's what's expected of us: We are supposed to always be on tap and interacting actively with our children. We aren't supposed to get

home from work and collapse for an hour, and then have to order a pizza because we just can't get dinner organized. Also, we aren't supposed to be messier than our toddler!
—Nora, 33, mother of a messy two-year-old child

In this section, I'll plunge into specifics for the "good" mom and then talk about how ADD moms stack up to this image. I'll call society's image "Ideal Mom."

In fact, I would love to hire Ideal Mom to come to my house and run everything! At first I thought she might be Mary Poppins or maybe Alice, the maid from the old TV show, "The Brady Bunch." But no, Ideal Mom is also employed full time at a great job, and she's a wonderful wife in addition to being Ideal Mom.

I wonder if anyone remembers an old TV commercial in which an attractive twenty-something woman sings about how she can come home from work and fry dinner up in a pan, take care of the kids, and never ever let you (her husband) forget you're a man! In other words, she's a hard worker, great mother, and sizzling sexual partner. And she cooks and cleans too. Who is this woman? She's the image we're all supposed to live up to. And we women with ADD are among the least likely to succeed.

Reliability: Doing What You're Supposed to Do, and on Time

Ideal Mom knows where everyone's sneakers are, she has the date and time of each appointment memorized, and she can throw together a perfectly balanced, nutritious meal in a jiffy—after working all day at the office. You can always count on Ideal Mom.

I recall reading that former TV host Phil Donahue once asked his wife, Marlo Thomas, where his shoes were. I loved her retort: "Where are *my* shoes?" Marlo was not "Mom" in this example, but her kind of thinking and her snappy comeback were a refreshing surprise to read about and also food for thought. Isn't it hard enough to keep track of your own things? Sure it is! Unless, of course, you are—Ideal Mom.

Self-Discipline: Following One Task Straight through to the End

Another important trait for mothers, as society sees it, is that Ideal Mom finishes what she starts, whether it's making three dozen cookies for the Cub Scouts meeting or ensuring her work responsibilities are fulfilled. In addition, she's the family manager, keeping track of everyone's schedule—the soccer practices, the music lessons, and the myriad events of life in the 21st century. Ideal Mom has a huge load of heavy expectations weighing her down. But she never lets it get her down.

Concentration: Ignoring Outside Distractions

Paying attention to what's going on around her is important, and Ideal Mom has no problem with this. The phone's ringing, the children are fighting, and there's an important report to finish tonight or her boss will be terribly upset. Ideal Mom calmly prioritizes everything in her head and accomplishes all tasks in her usual Ideal Mom-ish manner.

Self-Control: Maintaining Your Temper

Of course it's also important, or so the stereotype goes, for Mom to be ever serene, even in the face of extreme adversity. Even on one of "those days" when everything goes wrong. Does this sound familiar? You get up with a headache and things go straight downhill from there. A plumber agrees to come to solve a serious leak in the kitchen sink, and you stay home from work. Seven hours later, he's still not there.

And there's more. Your daughter's teacher calls to check if you made those five dozen cookies your child signed you up for—they're needed for the party tonight. Your daughter somehow forgot to tell you about this obligation she had committed you to. And one of the goldfish died and your little boy is heartsick. Flush it down the toilet? No way! He wants a burial in the backyard.

None of this is a problem for Ideal Mom! She'll take an aspirin for her headache, efficiently hire another plumber, and quickly bake up those cookies. Not only that, she arranges a funeral for Goldie the goldfish, to a tearful but mollified little boy's satisfaction. Gosh, how does she do it all? Don't be silly! She is Ideal Mom.

Parental Control over Children's Behavior

Once in awhile, Ideal Mom's children misbehave, ever so briefly. Not a problem. Ideal Mom swiftly disciplines them with the just-right technique, whether it's time-outs or charts with stars or whatever the latest magazine article says is *the* correct way.

And if the kids are tired or sick and are acting up because of it, Ideal Mom realizes this. She beams at disapproving strangers who frown at her crying children, explaining that they are "overtired" or not feeling well. She seems so wonderful that the frowns turn into grins as formerly crabby onlookers respond to her warmth.

Neatness: You Could Eat off Her Floor—Almost

Another aspect of Ideal Mom is that she is not only organized but she is also always very neat. Items are all put away in predictable places. The floors are uncluttered and the countertops are clear. You can't really eat off her floors—not that they aren't clean enough! But she just wouldn't let you. Good heavens, sit down at the table, please.

All the clothes in Ideal Mom's house are hung up or folded neatly in bureau drawers, unless they need to be washed. In that case, they are in a clothes hamper or a basket in the laundry room. Not just Mom's clothes, of course, but also her children's clothes. No stray socks, no clothes under beds. Ideal Mom wouldn't put up with that.

Tact and Diplomacy

Saying the right thing at the right time—a comforting word to an upset child or a firm correction to two children in an apparent death struggle over some minor toy—is an expected "Mom" skill, and one Ideal Mom has mastered. She can deftly defuse a spat between warring children or even angry adults. She should probably work for the State Department, she is that good. But no, she'd rather be Ideal Mom.

MAYBE YOU'RE NOT AS GOOD AS YOUR MOTHER WAS!

But, did your mother—

- Have a full-time, paying job? (probably not)
- Expect her earnings to count for a significant part (or all) of the family support?
- Believe she could quit at any time?
- Help with homework every night? (many parents today are expected to do this)
- Have neighbors, relatives, and friends she could rely upon for help?
- Have to worry about promotions or pay raises?

▶ MOMS WITH ADD: WHAT THE WORLD USUALLY GETS

"I was beaten into submission when I was a girl. I did not look hyper for the most part in school but my mind and my limbs were always going a mile a minute."
—Diane, 44, mother of an eight-year-old son with ADD

By now it should be apparent that I believe even most non-ADD moms cannot achieve this wonderful, mystical ideal and are often very frustrated in the face of these unreasonable expectations. It's even harder for the mom with ADD. She's disorganized, forgetful, and exhibits other traits of ADD—she's an easy target when we're stacking up moms against Ideal Mom.

"Real" non-ADD mom may not behave perfectly. She can't be as good as the ideal, but *at least* she's better than that mother with ADD over there. In turn, the mom with ADD is beating herself up mentally because she can't meet the ideal *or* the achievements of the non-ADD mom.

It's not that she doesn't love her children; she does. But no matter how hard she tries, it's impossible to evolve into the image that others—and she herself—have set as the one right way to be. As a result of this apparent shortfall, moms with ADD can develop very low self-esteem, grafted onto the low self-esteem problem that stems from childhood criticisms and slights. To illustrate the problem in its elements, let's take a look at what many moms with ADD are really like.

Losing Track of Time: Is Today Monday or Tuesday? It's February, Right?

A hallmark of attention deficit disorder is difficulty with organization, so the mom with ADD is inherently disadvantaged at achieving the high level of organization that society sees as normal and good for all mothers. The mother with ADD often loses items, and sometimes she forgets to accomplish tasks that other people are counting on her to perform.

If it were not for my watch and my calendar, I would often forget what day it is— so thank goodness for these tools! When you have ADD, time isn't necessarily linear—with one day stopping and then a brand-new day starting. Instead, time seems either like *now* or like one continuous, surging-ahead process. You know time is moving forward, of course. But often when you are actively working on different projects, as many of us are, it's easy to lose track of time. And, as I'll discuss in Chapter Two, "Zeroing in on the Good Aspects of ADD," many moms with ADD can hyperfocus, which means they concentrate so intently that they completely lose track of time as hours speed on by them.

Forgetting Things:
I Just *Know* There's Something I'm Supposed to Do Today

Did you ever put something in a special place where it would be "safe"—and then forget where that was and never find the object again? It happens to just about everyone, but it happens much more frequently to the mom with ADD. The world expects Ideal Mom to be the repository/human computer of the schedule of every single family member. But often the mom with ADD has trouble remembering what she herself is supposed to be doing, let alone what everyone else's schedule is.

Being Impulsive: Quick-Change Artists at Decision-Making

Another key feature of ADD is impulsiveness—your thought and act are almost simultaneous. You see something off the road that interests you, so you go look at it, even though you are supposed to be at your sister's house in fifteen minutes.

Ideal Mom doesn't have a problem with this. If she's supposed to be somewhere, she makes darn sure she does everything possible to be there, and on time.

Non-ADD Mom, who is human though not ideal, generally can make a plan and be on time. She is not easily distracted by sights, sounds, or her own thoughts that stimulate her while driving to her destination. Non-ADD Mom screens out what she considers irrelevant and is able to do so mostly unconsciously. But the mom with ADD often has trouble sorting out many interesting items and events. If something more interesting suddenly appears on her mental radar screen, she is likely to pursue that exciting new opportunity and temporarily forget about her original plans.

Losing Important Items: Where's That School Permission Form?

Many mothers with ADD say they drive themselves crazy with the things they lose: their car keys, papers they need, school permission forms, and so on. One good thing about looking for lost things: While you're frantically looking for a lost item, you often find other things that were long ago given up for dead, and you briefly rejoice at your findings before returning to the search.

Many of us are so easily distracted, we forget that we resolved to put the car keys on the table, or the purse on the chair—or the whatever, wherever. Whatever is distracting us is drawing us in, and the car keys and purse are forgotten and go wherever they happen to be laid down or dropped.

An unsolvable problem? Certainly not. One way to engrain a new good habit is to "overlearn" it. For example, putting your purse precisely in the same place, every time. After awhile, it becomes automatic.

Katie always checks her purse before leaving a place to make sure her keys are in there. Sometimes she double-checks. She said that one psychiatrist (pre-ADD diagnosis) told her that she definitely had "obsessive-compulsive disorder" because of all this checking. He wouldn't listen when she explained to him that after losing her keys so many times, she'd finally had enough. She was going to solve the problem. And she has: Since starting the planned key checking, she hasn't lost her keys.

Katie didn't listen to the OCD-obsessed doctor and found another psychiatrist who easily diagnosed her ADD. And he complimented her on her coping tactics too!

Procrastinating: Today, Tomorrow, Whatever

Many ADDers have a problem with delaying tasks for so long that they miss deadlines, are late for appointments, or have to rush to get things done at the last minute. It's not that they are lazy or don't want to do these things. It's just that for many, their sense of time is *now* and *later*. And later doesn't matter.

Being Blunt: You Don't Have to Wonder How ADD Moms Feel

"My opinions often tumble out. It has been difficult to curb my own abrasiveness," said Jackie, 29, mother of one. Many moms with ADD have difficulty with holding their tongues when around their family, friends, or fellow workers, when it would be better to think before speaking.

It's not that the person blurting out a comment means to be cruel, outrageous, or tactless, or just plain not nice. What happens is that she just says what everyone else may be thinking—but not saying. Maybe Aunt Sally really *is* too chubby to be wearing a purple polka-dotted dress tied with a huge sash; and okay, maybe *others* might think she looks like a large, garish birthday present. They probably won't say it. But the mom with ADD may say exactly what is on her mind—and watch out, Aunt Sally.

Coping with Messiness: Clutter, Clutter Everywhere

One common problem many of us face is the massive clutter that seems to constantly reproduce itself everywhere. Ideal Mom would be revolted by such chaos.

In fact, the mom with ADD may ask herself, how did we end up with so much *stuff*? If you really want to know, here's the answer: While you're not looking, tiny gremlins are coming out of corners and piling up more useless stuff, at the same time stealing one each of many pairs of socks and shoes. It's all their fault.

Of course, that is not it. Clutter accumulates because we bring home more stuff and don't get rid of already-existing items, including many we don't need. Another problem: The more junk you amass, the harder it is to get rid of even part of it, because the cleanup job looks so huge as to seem impossible.

Disciplining Kids: Dazed and Confused

Catch an ADD mom out with her child in public during a meltdown-level temper tantrum, and you may well see a woman with eyes glazed over, looking like she doesn't quite know where she is. Or she may be yelling at the child, acting nearly as childish as the tired three-year-old. Ideal Mom would never act this way. But the mom with ADD, overtired and overstressed, sometimes may well feel like she's losing it.

Of course, parents don't get special rulebooks or manuals when babies are born. And no matter how many parenting classes they take or how many self-help books by expert pediatricians they read, it's still a very tough job for every parent.

The mom with ADD may become so frustrated and confused that she will use bribery (such as the candy bar she grabbed from the checkout counter aisle), threats, or just about anything else—all to disapproving stares of onlookers—to stop the child's yelling and end the agony.

MOMS WITH ADD ANSWERED THIS QUESTION: IF YOU COULD MAKE A MAGIC WISH RELATED TO YOUR ADD (AND CAN'T WISH IT GONE), WHAT WOULD YOU WISH?

- For people to understand I don't have to be a walking calendar to be a wonderful person.

- That I could harness the energy, creativity, intensity, and sometimes brilliance—and drive it like one of those high-performance cars. Once in awhile my medication gives me the incredible sensation of running on all cylinders.

- That I could just say what I mean instead of talking in circles to get there and then keeping some important parts of what I am trying to say inside my head.

- That I could be less hard on myself.

- That I had a link to my hard drive while I sleep, so I could download all the creative thoughts that come to me at night when I sleep.

- That schools and workplaces would readily accommodate people with ADD.

- That I could be happy with days when nothing out of the ordinary happens. Usually I think the day was wasted if I didn't learn anything new.

- That the people I am closest to were as interested in ADD as I am and would educate themselves thoroughly.

- I wish my children's father believed it existed at all.

- That I could steer my ADD son through school to avoid the scars school left on me.

- I wish I could direct all my wonderful energy toward focused behaviors at will.

Focusing: Some ADD Moms Are Easily Distracted

"I feel as though I live from one interruption to the next. The problem is, each interruption takes me away from a task and I leave a trail of unfinished things behind me."
—Shannon, age 38, mother of two school-age sons.

"If you keep getting interrupted, mostly by your own shifting mass of thoughts and impulses, and as a result it takes 4½ hours instead of 55 minutes to bake a cake, how can you hope to get perfectly decorated cupcakes to the classroom in time for your child's birthday party? Beyond that, it's a challenge to listen, be attentive, not finish other people's sentences for them, and help your child be organized when you're an organizational disaster yourself," says Judy, 44, mother of one daughter.

Being Hyperactive: I Can't Sit Still

Some mothers with ADD also experience hyperactivity—what we used to call "ants in the pants." She can't sit still, she's always on the go; but because of her ADD, she doesn't get a whole lot accomplished. Of course, this high energy level is not always a curse. Many hyperactive moms have learned to harness and control this hyperactivity beast, much like taming a bucking bronco.

Jennifer, 29, the mother of a school-age son and daughter, says, "When I was in grade school, my only friends were boys. Girls didn't like me. I played Army with the boys and we used to dig tunnels through the snow. One day, some of my friends and I got some old sheets and cut them into smaller squares. We tied them into the shape of parachutes and jumped off the townhouses on the base. The snow was at least four or five feet deep where we were jumping.

"Some of the parents thought it was cool until they suddenly discovered I was not a boy. Everyone freaked when they found out I had actually jumped off the townhouse roof with the boys. Girls aren't supposed to do those things. Or so I was told."

IS SOCIETY MORE ACCEPTING OF MEN AND BOYS WITH ADD?

Many of my interviewees said boys and men got the better deal on this one.

- Boys are expected to be rough and tumble. Girls are not.
- Women with ADD are seen as stupid or lazy. Men may be seen as stubborn.
- People associate ADD with bad behavior. Since most women are just daydreamers, it's assumed they are lazy or dippy.
- People think boys must have a medical problem. But girls are "flighty."
- It's okay to be an absent-minded professor if you're a man. Not if you are a woman.
- People seem to expect males *not* to think before they act, because "Boys will be boys." Not so for girls.
- It's easier for men to be diagnosed and expect the world to make accommodations. Women are supposedly "born" accommodaters.
- Men are generally not seen as the organizing agent of family, household, and children.
- It is seen as more OK for boys to act rambunctiously than girls.

Yet it does not have to be that way. We can't change the unrealistic view our society holds of the way moms should be, including perfectly balancing a tough day on the job with exquisite "quality time" with the kids.

What can change is the way that ADD moms regard themselves. They can also incorporate coping mechanisms into their behaviors that enable them to cope better.

Living with ADD: An Explanation, Not an Excuse

A key point to remember if you or someone else you care about has ADD is that it is a diagnosis and an explanation. It is not an excuse or an exemption from most of life's requirements, although certainly accommodations can and should be made. Sometimes unbelievers think that we are trying to "get out of" our obligations. The fact is, most of us are doing our utmost to fulfill them.

This ADD mom hopes that you will find the information in this book liberating and helpful, and that you will walk away from reading it with a new, positive sense of yourself and the possibilities that lie ahead. Knowledge is power!

▶ **HOW EXPERTS DIAGNOSE ADD**

The diagnostic "bible" of psychiatrists and therapists is the *Diagnostic and Statistical Manual of Mental Disorders: DSM-IV,* published by the American Psychiatric Association in 1994. This book covers everything from "caffeine-related disorders" to very serious illnesses such as schizophrenia, bipolar disorder (manic depression), and others. Psychiatrists view a sort of menu of symptoms, and if a patient has more than a certain number from the list, then she may be diagnosed with the disorder.

When it comes to ADD, or, as the *DSM-IV* calls it, "attention-deficit hyperactivity disorders," the three primary features are inattention, hyperactivity, and impulsivity. (You can have attention disorder without hyperactivity, however.)

Here are some excerpts from the *DSM* about how inattention is defined:

> "Inattention may be manifest in academic, occupational, or social situations. Individuals with this disorder may fail to give close attention to details or may make careless mistakes in schoolwork or other tasks. Work is often messy and performed carelessly and without considered thought. Individuals often have difficulty sustaining attention in tasks or play activities and find it hard to persist with tasks until completion.

> "They [those with ADD] often appear as if their mind is elsewhere or as if they are not listening or did not hear what has just been said. There may be frequent shifts from one uncompleted activity to another. Individuals diagnosed with this disorder may begin a task, move on to another, then turn to yet something else, prior to completing any one task.

> "Work habits are often disorganized and the materials necessary for doing the task are often scattered, lost, or carelessly handled and damaged. Individuals with this disorder are easily distracted by irrelevant stimuli and frequently interrupt ongoing tasks to attend to trivial noises or events that are usually and easily ignored by others. They are often forgetful in daily activities (e.g., missing appointments, forgetting to bring lunch).

> "In social situations, inattention may be expressed as frequent shifts in conversation, not listening to others, not keeping up one's end of conversations, and not following details or rules of games or activities."

In case you're wondering, references to *play* and forgetting to bring your lunch are really for children with ADD; doctors use the same guidelines for children and adults.

As mentioned, another feature of ADD may be hyperactivity. Although women seem to exhibit hyperactivity less frequently than do men who have ADD, many of the women I interviewed were clearly hyperactive.

Another major feature of ADD is impulsivity. The *DSM* says, "Individuals with this disorder typically make comments out of turn, fail to listen to directions, initiate conversations at inappropriate times, interrupt others excessively, intrude on others."

Professional Experience

Psychologists and psychiatrists also ask many questions, and based on their own knowledge and experience, decide whether a person has ADD.

Note: To know for sure if you have ADD, a psychologist, psychiatrist, or therapist must diagnose you. Don't leave your choice of a doctor or therapist to chance, or you could end up with an incompetent person. Read Chapter Thirteen, "Professional Help."

Note on Terminology

The *DSM-IV* uses *attention deficit disorder with hyperactivity* to denote ADD that is primarily the "inattentive" type as well as the hyperactive form. Thus, if you are mostly inattentive, you have attention deficit hyperactivity disorder—without hyperactivity. Hyperactive but no hyperactivity? Frankly, I don't get it. As a result, I am using the phrase "attention deficit disorder" or "ADD" to encompass both forms.

▶ **SARI SOLDEN SCREENING CHECKLIST FOR WOMEN WITH ADD**

This checklist, developed by therapist and author Sari Solden, is quite fascinating and can be very revealing for readers. It is a list of characteristics that tend to predict whether a person has ADD. Everyone has these kinds of feelings at some time and to some extent. Do you have them more severely? Have they been present for most of your life? Are they giving you an overwhelming sense of difficulty in achievement, self-esteem, relationships, and mood?

❏ **Do you feel bombarded in department stores, grocery stores, at the office, or at parties?**

❏ **Do you often shut down in the middle of the day, feeling assaulted?**

❏ **Is time, money, paper, or "stuff" dominating your life and impacting your ability to achieve your goals?**

❏ **Are you spending a majority of your time coping, looking for things, catching up, or covering up?**

❏ Are you avoiding people because of all of this, hiding big chunks of yourself out of shame?

❏ Have you stopped having people over to your house because of your shame at the mess?

❏ Even though you are educated, have you never learned to balance your checkbook?

❏ Is it impossible for you to shut out nearby sounds and distractions that don't bother others?

❏ Do small requests for "one more thing" put you over the top emotionally?

❏ Do you often feel life racing out of control, that it's impossible to meet demands?

❏ Do you start out each day determined to get organized?

❏ Do you feel like a couch potato or tornado, at either end of the activity spectrum?

❏ Do you feel that you have many more ideas than others, but you can't stop them or synthesize, organize, or act on them in a orderly way?

❏ Have you watched others of equal IQ and education pass you by?

❏ Are you starting to feel despair of ever fulfilling your potential and meeting your goals?

❏ Are you clueless as to how others lead a consistent, regular life?

❏ Have you been thought of as selfish because you don't write thank-you notes or send birthday cards? Are you called a slob or spacey? Are you "passing for normal"? Does it feel more and more as if you were an imposter?

❏ Is all your time and energy taken up with coping, staying organized, holding it to-gether, with no time for fun or relaxation?

In this chapter, I have defined key problems faced by mothers with ADD and compared the way society expects mothers to act (Ideal Mom) to the way moms with ADD often do act. The chapter also explores why some people have trouble accepting that ADD even exists and concludes with a self-test for the person who wonders if she may have ADD.

2

Zeroing in on the Good Aspects of ADD

I never knew until the day I told my mother I was diagnosed with ADD that she had always blamed *herself* for problems I had as a child. She started crying, just from sheer relief of knowing it wasn't her fault at all. It wasn't my fault either. It was just ADD.
—Amy, 39, mother of two children

I think it's really important for ADD moms to forgive themselves for not being "Supermom." My basic theory about being a parent is you do the best you can and that is all you CAN do.

"It was a major shock for me when I realized that the boring, slow people were the normal ones," says Lois, 45 and mother of two sons. "I just couldn't believe it at first!" Lois has a very positive mental attitude about her ADD and the benefits it brings to her. In fact, many women with ADD have successfully harnessed the good parts of ADD.

Some psychologists see ADD in black-and-white terms only. But there are some advantages to ADD, and many women with ADD are highly intelligent and creative people. They have a "different kind of brain." As a result, although there are many problems when you are a mom with ADD, I decided to accentuate the positive in this chapter and then move on to "Working on Solutions to Common ADD Problems" (Chapter Three).

The key positive features of ADD covered in this chapter are

> **Hyperfocusing**
> **Curiosity**
> **Creativity and spontaneity**
> **Compassion, sensitivity, and empathy**
> **Sense of humor**
> **High energy**
> **Living in the now**
> **Commitment to children**
> **Multitasking ability**

Other positive features are a compassion and sensitivity for the difficulties of others. This may seem paradoxical in the face of the rather harsh description I quoted from the *DSM-IV* in Chapter One. And yet, although people with ADD may be inattentive, impulsive, and/or hyperactive, their ability to see many details can sometimes make them acutely sensitive. Further, because most people with ADD have suffered from a great deal of criticism, they know what it feels like to be the underdog.

▶ HYPERFOCUSING

I can surf the Web for hours without taking a single break.
—Judy, 39, mother of one son

Do you hyperfocus? Maybe, if you see yourself in these scenarios:

- I can work on the computer 4–5 hours straight. I may not have eaten all day because I'm focusing on a subject. The house is dirty and the dinner needs to be cooked.
- I can work in the garden for hours, not stopping for anything, and getting things squared away at a level of detail that is unusual for me.
- I design database systems and decorate cakes. I can spend countless hours on either of these tasks—so long as my glass of Diet Pepsi is kept full for me.
- I get so engrossed in what I'm doing that the world goes away for awhile. Once I have pulled my focus together, it's very hard to pull it away, and interruptions make me very upset.

Another woman who can hyperfocus for hours is Laura, 31, and parent to one son. One day she decided to make her son an afghan cover for his bed, readied her yarn and utensils and began. She finally stopped working six hours later, which seemed to Laura to be about five minutes. She had lost all track of time in her blinders-on dedication and fascination to performing the tasks involved in making that afghan for her son.

Many people with ADD report that they can spend long periods of time on activities that interest them—in fact, much longer periods than most non-ADD people will spend. This can be a plus if you are working on a job that needs to be done quickly and requires intense concentration. It can also be a minus—for example, if a mother gets too wrapped up in a project and forgets to perform an important task. This is easy to do!

Despite the problems it can bring when unharnessed, I think the ability to hyperfocus is the greatest gift my ADD gives me and many others. I like the ability to concentrate very intensely for four or five hours straight. In fact, I think hyperfocusing is akin to the concept of "flow" that some scientists have described: As you work on a project, you move seamlessly from one task to the next and the next, feeling completely confident at what you are doing. You feel "as one" with the task. It may sound mystical, but flow—and hyperfocusing—are by-products of an intensely creative mind.

Oftentimes you may know that you are hyperfocusing while in the middle of a project and feel it's okay. Or you may not notice your behavior until hours later, when you think, "I did all that in just five hours? That's amazing."

It's good when the mom with ADD acknowledges what she's achieved through hyperfocusing. The bad part comes when, instead of acknowledging her creation, she says, "How come most of the time I can barely think to come in out of the rain, I lose my car keys at least weekly, and I haven't balanced my checkbook in months?" Moms who think only of the negatives need to balance more than their checkbooks; they need to balance their self-assessments too.

TERRY MATLEN IS A MICHIGAN THERAPIST WHO SPECIALIZES IN COUNSELING WOMEN WITH ADD. HERE'S WHAT SHE HAS TO SAY ABOUT THE POSITIVES.

ADD can interfere greatly with daily activities and damage self-esteem. But every client I have worked with has also had amazing gifts. Though the research so far may not support what I see in my office, most adults with ADD seem to be more compassionate, sensitive, creative, and humorous. They also have a knack for finding novel solutions to problems!

Many do come in with years of negative self-talk in their vocabularies, failures in school and work experiences and in relationships as well. I remind them they excel in areas others may have difficulties in. I encourage them to take the next step in whatever venture they hope to accomplish, with their new understanding of how their own brand of ADD affects them. With therapy, education, medication, and coaching, ADD adults can make wonderful life changes.

▶ **CURIOSITY**

Based on my interviews and observations, another positive trait shared by many moms with ADD is an intense curiosity. They report a variety of interests and a need to know more, more, more. Curiosity is a trait that can be used to great advantage as a mom! When other moms stop asking questions, the ADD mom can think of many more issues to ask about—and to convince her child to think about. She can also see problems from different angles, and she's adept at coming up with several possible solutions.

Once when my son was about three years old and a little whiney from a cold, I told him he was going to learn something about the scientific method. No, I didn't read him a bunch of medical journal articles or rush out and spend $200 on computer programs or the latest toy recommended by child psychologists. Instead, I told him I wondered how fast ice would melt. Would it melt faster in the shade or the sun? We should investigate. Being very curious himself, my son was eager to know what would come next.

Of course, I knew ice in the sun would melt fast, but didn't actually know *how* fast. So we went outside with ice cubes and a stopwatch, discussing our "hypothesis" and method. I showed him how the stopwatch worked. We pondered the exact placement of our ice cubes and then set one ice cube in a sunny spot and another in the shade.

It was a warm day and we didn't have to wait long. I timed each ice cube while my son watched in rapt attention, running back and forth between them and telling me "Now!" when the ice cube was no longer solid. Then he suggested different kinds of shade, darker and lighter and other variations. We retrieved more ice cubes and did more experiments. I let him use the stopwatch and I said "Now!" I wrote down our results and we discussed what it all meant.

I told my son that he was a scientist and I was very proud of him! I thought then—and still think—learning can be sheer joy, although others often make it boring. Even frozen water can be intriguing! I guess I feel that way because my son and I are curious people, as are many people with ADD.

▶ **CREATIVITY AND SPONTANEITY: NONLINEAR THINKING**

I'm great at bouncing ideas around, so long as I don't have to remember them. I can be a very good idea catalyst for people.
—Petra, 27, mother of a toddler son

Creativity is another common feature of people with ADD. If you want someone who can envision many different ways to do a job—or have fun—the mom with ADD is often the right person. Her nonlinear brain frequently enables her to think beyond going from just point A to point B. Instead, she can leap off from point A all the way to point Q, then to point Z and back again—while most people are still ponderously on their way to point B.

Of course, the mom with ADD might not always be the best person to decide which course of action is the right one, and she might be the worst person to make sure the plan is followed once started. But if people give ADD Mom a chance, they can gain a great deal in the form of wonderful ideas.

"I get quite a lot of ideas other people find strange but they make my life easier," says Ann, 35, mother of one son. "A good example is the kitty litter problem. My dogs liked to invade the litter box, which really upset the cat. I bought a toddler gate and cut a hole just big enough for the cat to squeeze through. I put the litter box in a closet and fit the gate to the doorway. Now the cat has her own private space where the dogs can't get to her. And I saved money on cat litter!"

Isn't creativity the same as curiosity, another trait we just discussed? I don't think so, although I believe the curious person is often creative too. The difference is that you can be curious about a subject but not make any inroads into solving a particular problem. Creative people are curious but they are also problem-solvers.

"The workforce calls it 'thinking outside the box.' Having and/or living with someone with ADHD forces you to examine tired-out premises and question and challenge the status quo," said Deanna, 32, mother of two schoolage children.

Society Doesn't Always Appreciate Creative People

Creativity isn't always valued. Creative people can be annoying to others. They often challenge and annoy others who insist the world is flat. They may also get in the way and not give up when they think they're on the track of some great discovery. They may not be good "team players" and may operate outside the structure needed by others.

In an article for the *Journal of Creative Behavior*, Bonnie Cramond described her research and speculations on a link between creativity and attention deficit disorder in children. She also described the daydreaming and impulsivity of great thinkers and inventors and the difficulty they had in school.

Cramond tested children with ADD and found them highly creative. She also found that routine, quiet, and structure was usually recommended for such children, although it was ineffective for them, at best. Instead, such children needed *less* structure, not more. In fact, their creativity could easily be stifled by rigid structure. One child with the inattentive form of ADD tested in the 99th percentile for creativity. Cramond said:

> The recommendations for Benjamin included breaking down verbal directions into simple steps, and emphasizing structure and routine in the classroom. These are standard recommendations for children who are diagnosed as suffering from ADHD, however, they are anathematic for a creative, sensation-seeking child. These recommendations, if applied to such children, might partly explain the poor results that have been noted in treating children labeled ADHD.

What about creative adults? They too come up with brilliant, off-the-wall ideas, and they also often fill out their travel vouchers incorrectly and forget to file them on time. Do they remember to punch in—or out? Probably not.

As a result, creativity is an asset of many children and adults with ADD, but it's not always appreciated. However, if anyone is able to appreciate creativity in her child, with ADD or not, who's better than a mom with ADD? We have a built-in parenting plus.

Creativity Smashers and Boosters

It's important to carefully nurture our own creativity as well as that of our children. Creativity can be stimulated or it can be inhibited, and often moms with ADD are so down on themselves that the inhibition choice is more likely. Yet most of us learn from our mistakes. The famous inventor Thomas Edison (who may have had ADD) said, "I didn't fail ten thousand times. I successfully eliminated, ten thousand times, materials and combinations which wouldn't work."

Here is a list of possible "creativity smashers" and "creativity propellers":

Creativity Smashers	Creativity Boosters
Thinking, "I'm not smart enough to figure this out."	Telling yourself, "This is a tough problem. What are some possible solutions?"
Making a mistake and beating yourself up over it.	Making a mistake and thinking "How can I correct this?" and "How can I do this differently next time?"
Keeping the same routine, every day.	Trying something different: a new way home, a new food, etc. Taking a shower if you always take baths (or baths, if you always take showers).

Spontaneity/Impulsivity

The mom often criticized for her sudden, impulsive actions may find herself admired in some circumstances. She may be adept at solving problems occurring right now—problems that could paralyze a non-ADD woman who is primarily future oriented.

"When there's an emergency, I just do what needs to be done. I don't think of consequences and don't worry about who might be offended. I just act and right away," says Mara, 41, mother of an 11-year-old girl.

► COMPASSION, SENSITIVITY, AND EMPATHY

I think it's important for mothers with ADD to model interdependence and teach their children that sometimes you need help. We all have

gaps. A child could get a partner for a project. Use your strengths to direct your creativity or sensitivity.
—Sari Solden, author of *Women with Attention Deficit Disorder*

Although the mom with ADD may be a very blunt person who blurts out statements before she thinks, many ADD moms are also very caring and compassionate people. They know from experience what it's like to be the odd person out, the one not chosen for the team, and the one perceived as not part of the regular group.

"I have found over and over again in twenty years of working with 'funny brains' (ADD, learning disabled and mild head injury) that these people are more compassionate than others. They *know* what it is like to have a weakness, yet be smart. They *know* what it is like to be criticized for faults they cannot seem to correct. They know so many of the frailties that beset humans, because they know it from the inside," said James Lawrence Thomas, Ph.D., author of *Do You Have Attention Deficit Disorder?* (Dell, 1996).

Laura, 33 and mother of a 10-year-old boy, agrees and says, "When my son or I are having a bad day and nothing seems to work, we know it's just an ADD day.

"One day, I bought myself a cup of coffee and placed it on the car seat. I suddenly realized I had forgotten something, so I rushed into the store and came right back. And sat right down on a full cup of coffee. *That* is an ADD day kind of thing."

▶ SENSE OF HUMOR

I like my own silly sense of humor and my ability to laugh at myself. I'm amazingly adaptable since I've had lots of experience in trying to work myself out of disasters! Now that I know it's the way my brain works, I can accept myself. I'm still not like everybody else is. But I don't want to be like everybody else anymore.
—Sue, 34, mother of three sons ages 4, 7, and 11

Another asset possessed by many of us moms with ADD is a great sense of humor. An ability to see the lighter side in many things can make life easier for you and your children.

Humor Can Be a Great Distraction

Humor is often a great distraction to a cranky child, who may well find it hard not to laugh about Mom being so silly. I have stopped my child cold in the middle of a temper tantrum by making a ridiculous face or saying something off the wall. I'm not sure if it's the distraction or the humor involved, but humor can definitely be an anger-buster.

It can also break through to the school-age or teenage child who responds to everything you ask him with an "I don't know," or "I guess so," and similar noncommital remarks. One day Arlene, 46, in frustration with receiving these kinds of answers from her teenage son, said to him, "What are you going for here? Gandhi? Is this passive resistance to the Evil Parent?"

Her son was startled and laughed. The stalemate was over, and some real communication between them could begin.

ON THE LIGHTER SIDE: SPONTANEITY DEFICIT DISORDER

Psychologist and ADD expert Kathleen Nadeau used her creativity and humor to devise this checklist for diagnosing "spontaneity deficit disorder." Use it with non-ADD people who accentuate the downside of ADD. Have them answer yes or no to each question.

Spontaneity Deficit Disorder Checklist*

1. I find that sorting and folding socks is a deeply satisfying activity.

2. It's hard for me to think of new ideas, but I'm good at doing what I'm told.

3. I plan what I do, and I do what I plan.

4. I know how to spell *spontaneity,* but I'm not sure what it means.

5. As a child, I colored inside the lines.

6. I consider being called a linear thinker a compliment.

7. I'm good at filling out forms.

8. Checking items off my to-do list gives me a great feeling of accomplishment.

9. Unexpected events make me feel uncomfortable.

10. I keep all my ducks in a row.

If you answered yes to five or more items, you should probably seek an evaluation for spontaneity deficit disorder.

Above all, don't despair. There is value in being neat, orderly, and predictable. By working with a career counselor who specializes in treating spontaneity deficit disorder, you will be able to find an appropriate job or career path in which details and paperwork production are emphasized.

*Reprinted with permission of Kathleen G. Nadeau, Ph.D., Co-Editor, *ADDvance Magazine, A Magazine for Women with Attention Deficit Disorder.* This checklist first appeared in *ADDvance* (www.addvance.com).

Target your humor to your child's age and level of understanding. Silly puns might not be understood at all by small children and only groaned at by your teenagers—whereas a 10-year-old could find them hilarious.

Use Shared Humorous Events from Your Family History

You can also use humor based on your shared history as a family. For example, several years ago, my daughter was dating a new boy we didn't know well. He didn't have a car and she met him at the mall. Later, my husband and I were to pick her up after a party. She gave us directions but when we arrived, we found no sign of her.

**If I could remember your name, I'd ask if you've
seen my keys.**
—Anonymous comment by a person with ADD.

I ASKED MOMS WITH ADD: WHAT SURPRISED YOU THE MOST ABOUT ADD?

- How we compensate in order to appear "normal."
- My ADD has allowed me to be sillier than other moms I know, so I can enjoy being with the kids in a very different way than other moms can.
- Finding out there was a name for the way I was and a reason for it.
- How long I have survived!
- That my need to write down everything has a name.
- I thought it was just for hyperactive kids. I have the inattentive kind of ADD.
- That there are many others just like me.

Every possible bad thing that might have happened to her occurred to us, including ridiculous ones like the fear that she'd been sold into white slavery. You can get pretty paranoid on a dark night when you can't find someone you love.

My husband and I complained bitterly about *where* she was, and *what* were we going to do, and wasn't this awful? Our preteen son suddenly piped up from the back seat. "But Mom and Dad, don't you want to have an *adventure*?"

My husband and I looked at each other and burst out laughing. To us, this was an ordeal, but to our son, it was high adventure. "No! We didn't want an adventure, but we got one anyway!" I told him. We calmed down and moments later, found our daughter on the next street, outside a house and waiting for us. Sometimes when one of us complains a bit too much, my husband or I say, "Hey! Don't you want to have an adventure?" It usually defuses the situation.

▶ **HIGH ENERGY: WHEN THE ENERGIZER MOM KEEPS GOING AND GOING**

**As a mother, it's my job to interpret the world
for my kids and sometimes, okay most times, I**

don't do it the way the world would have me do it. It's not wrong, just different. There are many ways to get to a park. Just because society walks there doesn't mean someone else can't hop on a skateboard and get there just as well.
—Nora, 43, mother of two

Of course not all moms with ADD are hyperactive, but there are some who are very high-energy indeed. And a person with high energy can be seen not as hyperactive, but as highly enthusiastic, someone who can motivate everyone around her, is great at generating ideas, and "thinks on her feet."

▶ LIVING IN THE NOW

Although it can be a disadvantage at times, a "now" orientation can be an advantage too. While other people rush about, never seeing what's right before them and ever worried about next year or even ten years from now, the mom with ADD can appreciate her life and live "in the moment." She may not have a great future orientation but often the mom with ADD takes advantage of opportunities that exist right now—opportunities that another woman might turn down and later regret.

Not all moms with ADD have a joie-de-vivre approach to life, and for some, their inattentiveness tunes them out not only to next week but also to this minute. But for many, the ability to acutely feel and know they're alive now is a true asset.

▶ DEEP COMMITMENT TO CHILDREN

Many mothers with ADD are strongly committed to their children. This is a key reason why they feel such guilt and shame when their symptoms make it difficult or impossible to fulfill the role as well as they think they should.

"I wanted children so much and went through so much to get them—painful infertility treatments and counseling and worrying. And now sometimes they make me crazy! Which makes me feel guilty and confused because I really love them. The noise level could be hard to take," says Joanie, 38, mother of two daughters age five and seven.

Because of her deep commitment and love of her children, Joanie sought help and was diagnosed with ADD. She started taking medication and seeing a therapist to talk things out and now feels much more relaxed and happy with her family and her life. Of course, she is still not "Ideal Mom," as I described in Chapter One. But she is a loving and caring mother. She's a good mom.

▶ MULTITASKING ABILITY

Although some of us become confused by too much stimuli, many ADD moms are able to handle numerous tasks at the same time, if they're familiar with the jobs and they want to do them. You'll find these moms talking on the phone at the same time they're cooking dinner and checking on a child and thinking about what needs to be done tomorrow. Such moms may seem to others as if they have more arms than an octopus—and several brains as well!

This multitasking capability explains why many children with ADD are involved in many activities at once. My son can talk on the phone while watching television, eating a snack, and playing with the dog—and has no trouble juggling these tasks. But give him homework in more than two subjects, and watch out! Mass confusion.

Most people focus on the problematic aspects of ADD, but there are actually many positive aspects that we can mobilize to help us solve those problems. For example, many of us are creative, have a great sense of humor, and can multitask. In this chapter, I covered these positive elements and others common to the mom with ADD.

MYTHS AND REALITIES ABOUT MOMS WITH ADD

Myth: Women (and moms and girls) can't get ADD because it's a male thing.

Reality: Women and girls can have ADD. Experts have only recently begun to acknowledge this.

Myth: Females who have ADD aren't hyperactive.

Reality: Many girls and women seem more inattentive than hyperactive, but some are hyperactive.

Myth: If women with ADD tried harder, they could do as well as non-ADD women.

Reality: Women with ADD usually *are* trying harder. You can't give more than 100%.

Myth: Women with ADD can't be successful.

Reality: Many are successful, although it may be twice as hard for them as for the non-ADD person!

Myth: Women with ADD are terrible mothers.

Reality: Women with ADD may not be as neat and organized as their non-ADD counterparts. But they can be very good mothers.

3

Working on Solutions to Common ADD Problems

Sometimes it's just so difficult to get organized and to find so many lost things. Do you really think there's hope for us?
—Pam, 39, a mom with ADD who has three children

The answer is definitely yes, Pam! There are plenty of potential solutions to problems related to your ADD. No magical ones or perfect answers that make your ADD-related problems evaporate like fog before the sun. But there are practical ideas you can try to work on your problems—ideas that have worked for others.

This chapter discusses the following common problems many moms with ADD face. It also offers solutions that may work for you.

Getting organized
Losing things
Saying yes too much
Managing your time
Zoning out
Blurting out comments
Hyperreactivity to stimuli
High- and low-tech solutions

▶ LOST IN SPACE: ORGANIZATIONAL PROBLEMS AND SOLUTIONS

If you're like many mothers with ADD, you have a major problem with losing things. Maybe you forgot where you put them because you don't have one "special place" where important items like your keys are kept. Or maybe your items are so disorganized in the aggregate that you really did put those keys on your desk where you were supposed to place them—but there's so much clutter on top of the desk that you can't find them. Don't abandon hope. There are ways to resolve these problems.

Getting Started: Transforming Piles into Files

So where do you start, if you want to rid yourself of the chaos and become more organized? I'm not going to tell you that you have to give up *all* of your piles—I'm keeping a few of mine. But it's a good idea to limit the confusion.

Keep in mind that I can never tell you in one part of one chapter what experts have written entire books about. I recommend Georgene Lockwood's book on organizing. It's packed with info and fun to read: *The Complete Idiot's Guide to Organizing Your Life* is the definitive organizing book in my view. My goal is to get you jump-started.

The first thing you usually need to do is go through your papers. Separate personal papers from your work/business papers to minimize confusion, unless it's important to you to keep everything together in a central location. I pretend that work and personal papers are wildly allergic to each other and thus, they must be separated.

My personal checking account does not stay in my home office, nor are my birth certificate, children's birth certificates and other important papers located where I do my work. Instead, I recommend a metal, nonflammable box for your important personal papers—or a metal filing cabinet. Keep it in a safe place. If you keep work papers at home, I advise keeping them in a file cabinet or metal box as well.

A FEW MEMORY TRICKS

Do you have trouble remembering the names of items sometimes, or maybe a short list of what you were supposed to buy at the store? I do, as do many other people with ADD. (I tell my children it's because my brain is so crowded with information, that some of it spills over and gets lost.) Maybe you can use a few tricks that have helped me.

1. Associate the item with a visual image. I could not remember "quest planner," a special notebook my son uses in school. I could only remember it began with "q" and was always asking him if he had his "quality" thing. As I resolved to remember the correct name, the image of Don Quixote on his horse flashed into my head. Don Quixote was a character always on a quest. I imagined Quixote on his horse, lance facing outward. And stabbed through the end of his lance was—a quest planner! I never forgot the name again.

2. If you remember better by thinking of a sound, you could think of a song that reminds you of a word in the item, such as "The Impossible Dream," another quest theme.

3. If you need to remember short lists and forget to write them down (or forget the list itself), creating acronyms can help. Let's say I need milk, orange juice and peaches. I can think MOP—and also imagine a mop. I can also firm up the memory by thinking of bread that is sopping with milk, next to a glass of orange juice. Silly or unusual images are easier to remember. If I wanted to use a sound kind of memory aid, I could think of a song I remember from childhood, "Rag Mop," and mentally accentuate the MOP part.

Use your creativity to tailor memory tips to what works for *you*.

Next, go through your personal papers and divide them into three separate piles: important, maybe important, and I haven't used this in five or more years. If you have an accountant or tax advisor, ask her how long various financial items need to be kept, especially tax-related items. You will probably find that you don't need to go as far back as the papers that you do have! I recently threw away phone bills from 1985. Call the IRS and ask for IRS Publication No. 552 ("Recordkeeping for Individuals"), which tells you how long to keep documents related to taxes.

Then do the same thing for your work papers, separating them into important, maybe important, and really old stuff.

Here's the really hard part for most people with ADD: Throw away old, useless papers. The paperwork you still have on a car that you sold ten years ago is not important. A term paper you wrote twenty years ago is not important, even if you received an "A" on it! Throw it away! You may wish to buy an inexpensive paper shredder to rip up financial documents such as old canceled checks, so nobody can "dumpster dive" and find bank account numbers to use to their advantage.

After awhile, throwing out old stuff can be very liberating! Whether you run old canceled checks through an inexpensive paper shredder or rip them into shreds yourself, you create space and order out of chaos. In this case, destruction is actually constructive.

Don't Want to Give Up Your Piles?

Author Karen Jogerst (*If I Could Just Get Organized! Home Management Hope for Pilers & Filers*) divides the world into pilers and filers. Jogerst is a piler, and many women with ADD fall into this category. We like to *see* our things. We don't want them hidden in closed closets or bureau drawers—because then we forget about them.

Jogerst has suggestions for those who need their piles. For example, she sees containers as "tools, not luxuries," and relies on clear plastic containers that come in different sizes. Says Jogerst, "It is best to purchase containers for specific piles. You can get away with storing lightweight piles in cheaper ones, and so for things like children's clothing, extra pillows, and plasticware, cheaper brands work fine." For items such as books or camping gear, pay a little extra for a sturdier brand.

More Steps to Follow

Next, consider following these steps:

1. **Set up file categories you know you'll need.** Consider your needs and possible categories. For example, let's look at common household papers. You may be able to group them into the following categories:

- Receipts for tax-deductible items ("Tax Receipts")
- Bills to be paid ("Pay soon!")
- Bills you already paid ("Paid bills")
- Checking account statements ("Canceled checks')
- Credit card bills ("AmEx," "Visa," etc.)
- Legal items (your will, car titles, etc.)
- Important letters or faxes ("Needed letters/faxes")
- Contracts or warranties ("Written promises")

2. **Separate the papers in the work pile and personal file into categories.** Take the items from your "important" and "maybe important" piles. (You will have thrown out the old useless stuff by now!) Next, sort items into the categories you've selected. Some categories will "fit" both your personal and work lives, and some won't. For example, you may have a personal checking account but not a work checking account. You may have contracts with repairpersons in your personal life, but no contracts in your work life.

3. **Decide on additional categories you need.** Often after you've started organizing, you may discover items that don't fit any of the categories you've chosen. You can create a "miscellaneous" category, or if you have enough of these papers and they seem similar in some way, create a new category.

The Mail

I receive so much mail that for years I have been separating my mail into three piles. In fact, I try to sort the mail as soon as possible or certainly the same day—before it can run away and hide somewhere! I get a trash bag and set it next to me. In go the junk catalogs and ripped up credit card offers and solicitations I don't want.

If you get a lot of junk mail, throw it out. If it's a catalog you want, it isn't "junk" mail—because you want it. Make sure you rip up or shred any credit card offers that might include personal information those dumpster divers could use to defraud you with.

In some parts of the country, the approved method of disposing of junk mail is by recycling it, so you may need a special recycling bin for that purpose.

Moving on from Paper

Of course your clutter is not limited to papers and could well encompass a mind-boggling array of other items. As with the papers, you will also make three piles.

Only in this case, you start in one room, work for no more than two hours, then throw away the old junk. If you can't bear to throw it away and think it might be useful to someone, then give it to charity. And be realistic! Would a poor person really want or need this stuff?

Too Much Clutter

Remember this: Even when your house looks like a hurricane just hit it, you are still a beautiful child of the universe.

One major reason why so many of us ADD moms lose things is that there is too much clutter to look through to find the lost item. I think there are three primary reasons why ADD moms have an even tougher time with clutter than non-ADD moms: (1) you don't really see it; (2) if you do see it, it's a huge scary mess; and (3) you need a mindset shift.

1. **You don't really see it.** Seeing the problem is the first step toward solving it. But many of us ADD moms literally walk over it, around it, even underneath it—or on the ceiling—without seeing it.

When my mother enters a room, she can immediately see if and where things fit more efficiently. Not only that, she can also figure out—and fairly quickly—a better place for all the objects that seem out of place to her. This knack comes as easily to her as breathing, and she can't imagine not having such a skill. And I can't imagine what it would be like to have such a capability come naturally!

To understand what a person who doesn't have ADD sees when she enters a roomful of objects, it's something like this:

AAA	BBB	
CCC	DDD	EEE

But the same scene appears more like this to the person with ADD who has an organizational problem:

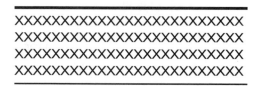

2. **If you do see it, it looks like a huge scary mess.** Even if we see the same items in about the same positions as the non-ADD person sees them, we

don't really *see* them, particularly as individual items contributing to the overall clutter. As a result, we who have trouble with clutter—even those of us with perfect vision—are more likely to see all the objects in a room as one huge blur. The items themselves don't have a cohesive pattern that is connected in our minds with a place.

Do you actually see the mess? Use this simple exercise to find out.

1. Walk into a major room of your house, say your living room or your bedroom.
2. Now, walk across the room in a straight line. Count the number of steps you can take before you encounter an object that does not belong there.
3. How many steps did you take?

Results

5+ steps: If you took five or more steps into the room, this is very good! The room may be messy, but it's safe and you probably can see the clutter.

3-4 steps: Good. Notice what you would be stepping over or tripping on when walking in a straight line. Where should those items really go?

1-2 steps: Yikes! Major clutter alert! The good news is that now you have a way to see and quantify the problems. And (hopefully) you are motivated to clear a path and do some serious clutter-busting.

When the non-ADD person sees a penny lying on the floor, she must pick it up and go put it in her penny holder. The mom with ADD picks it up and sets it aside someplace, almost immediately forgetting about it. She is not tying the item with the necessary place that the non-ADD person intuitively knows it *must* or *should* go to. And the mom with ADD is also often easily distracted—by the phone ringing or even a dog barking outside. She must go and investigate. The penny remains in the room and will probably fall on the floor again pretty soon.

How can you solve this problem? You can learn to emulate what a non-ADD person does and tailor it to your ADD needs, using your inherent creativity. One thing that non-ADD people do when they are picking up a room is they group items by where they should go in the house.

Let's say Anita, an ADD mom, is clearing the clutter in the living room. She has a good plan, which she is following. First, Anita picks up everything that doesn't belong in the living room. Then Anita groups items; for example, she places all items that should go into the bedroom in one group. Then she places all items that should go into the master bathroom in another group. If Anita finds any kitchen, garage, or other items, she makes more groupings of items.

The penny that Anita picked up goes with the quarter she also found, as well as with a dollar that fell out of a newly laundered pair of jeans. Incidentally, Anita had forgotten to check the pockets of the jeans before she washed them, and she's not alone. Many moms with ADD have plenty of "laundered money" in their homes because people forgot to take it out of their pockets before washing!

When she's finished picking up, Anita takes the items in the bedroom group to the bedroom. If she doesn't have time to put them away, she keeps them together in one place in the bedroom and does it later. Then she does the same with kitchen items, and so forth.

3. **You need a mindset shift.** Another major reason why many ADD moms have severe clutter problems is that we may have some wrongheaded ideas. What's needed is a shift in mindset, comprised of the following items: (a) understanding that jobs can be done in parts; (b) realizing that you shouldn't critique the job until you're done; (c) rewarding yourself for eliminating clutter; and (d) adopting clutter-busting as a goal for *you,* not your mom or the neighbors or the world.

- *Jobs can be done in parts.* As mentioned earlier, to the mom with ADD, clutter often looks like a huge blob of a problem because of her perception, as illustrated earlier. So she just leaves it there, whether it's an overflowing laundry basket of clothes, a pile of bills, or another mass of items that need attention.

  One of the secrets of organization is this: You don't have to do it all in one hour or one day. If you do a little bit at a time, then you will eventually get the clutter cleaned up. This means you can decide to attack the laundry today. Then, tomorrow or the next day, work on bills or another clutter that needs fixing.

  It's also a very good idea to spend no more than one or two hours on clutter-busting. Give yourself a realistic quota of time.

- *It isn't over until it's over: Don't critique the job until you're done.* Many moms with ADD start working on a project, and when they see they have *so much* left to do, they give up altogether. For this reason, withhold judgment on how you're doing until you are done. Unless you happen to notice that, wow! The room looks a *lot* better. Only positive self-comments are allowed.

  Here's another analogy. If a person needed to lose a lot of weight, let's say fifty pounds, wouldn't that seem horribly impossible? Think of the many negative things she might say to herself. Now consider another person. She too needs to lose fifty pounds, but instead of constantly beating herself up about it, or seeing she has *only* lost three pounds or *only* lost five pounds, she could say, "I'm going to lose five pounds."

  She puts the number in her mind and she works on it. When she has lost five pounds, she's happy and rewards herself, although not with food. Then, when she feels ready, she decides she'll lose another five pounds—or some other low amount. Eventually, she may or may not lose fifty pounds, but she is much more likely to lose weight than if she can see *only* the fifty-pound goal and nothing else.

Ridding your home of clutter is similar to the example of the woman needing to lose major weight. If you can see success *only* as a perfect home that looks like a photograph in a magazine, or *only* as a completely clear room, you'll get discouraged. Give yourself small, doable goals to achieve, so that most of the time, you can achieve them.

It's also important, as you clear the clutter, to realize that the mess is not *you*. It is just *stuff*. Powerless stuff! You are in charge. You will be the victor!

- *Rewards are important* Another crucial aspect is rewarding yourself. Self-rewards can be just as effective as the rewards you give to your children. After expending your clutter-busting time, you must reward yourself. Decide on the reward before you even start the job and then, when you've put in your one or two hours, give it to yourself.

   Make it a good reward, whether it's a trip to the bookstore or a very long bubble bath or something else you can look forward to. For example, Anita loves to go jogging by the park, so she resolves that after two hours of cleaning up the clutter in her living room, she is *owed* a jog that lasts as long as she feels like. Of course, the reward need not be athletic. Helen, who hates exercise, would shudder at the thought of jogging as a reward; but she could inspire herself with watching "General Hospital" and finding out what all those characters are up to today. Whatever works for you as a moderate reward is a good idea.

   When the job is totally done, it calls for an even better reward, say fifty laps around the park for Anita the jock or a tape of five shows for Helen.

TRASH BARRELS ARE GOOD

Don't try too hard to hide trash barrels because you think they're ugly —you might end up hiding them from yourself. Buy plastic trashcans in attractive colors, and place them in strategic points around your house: the kitchen, the family room, kids' rooms. Empty them at least once a week! Empty the kitchen trashcan daily.

For some of us, it is still very hard to throw items out, even when we know that we should do it and these things we are hanging onto aren't really important. If you have this problem, one strategy to try is the "halfway house" method. You put your probable throwaway items in a special place, such as the garage. You decide that in one week, you must make a final decision to throw these things out. You can also use the buddy system: Enlist the aid of a friend who will call you in one week and say, okay, it's Throwaway Junk Day! Time to get hopping!

- *Clutter-busting Is Achievable.* A lot of people think they should clear up the clutter in their house because their mother says they should, or because their neighbor thinks things are too messy. Or maybe they imagine that this mess would disgust the whole world.

The one person you need to empower is *you*. If you can envision eliminating clutter as simplifying your life and making things nice for you, and if you can imagine how much better it would be if things were not lost all the time, and you could walk straight through a room without tripping over skates or books, then you're on your way. See clutter-busting as a positive goal that you want to achieve for you, rather than an undoing of your evil ways. This mindset shift can make a very big difference!

After you've rid yourself of at least some of your clutter, you will have much less of a problem with losing things. However, don't assume that the problem is over forever!

▶ WHY AM I ALWAYS LOSING THINGS?

Do you have a problem with losing your keys, your money, your purse, and just about everything else? If you do, you have plenty of company! And no, this does not mean you have Alzheimer's disease at age 37. It may well be your ADD.

IT'S GOOD TO THROW STUFF OUT

Many Moms with ADD hate to throw anything away. You haven't worn that dress for fifteen years, but what if someday you go to Hawaii again and extremely flowered dresses are still popular there? Or maybe your daughter, age 3, would like it when she grows up.

If you don't want to throw it away, give it away to charity. And if it's not good enough for the Salvation Army, throw it *away*, girl! Along with all that other old junk you don't need anymore.

Experts say medication can help, and many women report that they lose things less often than before they began taking medication. They can focus better. But what if you still lose things? Here are some ideas for you.

Retracing Your Steps

If you lose a particular item, one simple tactic is to retrace your steps. You can try to think back, and you can actually visualize the path you followed around the time when you may have lost the item. Close your eyes and see what you saw then. It's okay to talk to yourself as you guide your way through this quick trip down recent-memory lane. Let me give an example.

To my horror one day, I discovered I had lost a check for $500. I searched my house and found nothing, nowhere. Then I panicked for a few minutes before I calmed down and used this method for retracing your steps:

1. **Think about the last time that you had the item.** For me, I remembered having the check after I retrieved it from the mail and took it inside the house. I put it inside my purse right away—so I wouldn't lose it.

2. **Think about everywhere you went after you knew that you had the item.** At first, I thought I had only been in the house. But then I remembered I'd also gone to the supermarket to buy a few items.

3. **Where were you, as precisely as you can remember?** I remembered where I parked in the parking lot, and I walked myself through the aisles of the supermarket in my mind, choosing the few items I needed.

4. **Go back.** I drove back to the supermarket and parked in the same spot. If I couldn't have parked there, I would have parked as near as possible. I walked in an increasing radius around the car and saw a few pieces of paper, but no! They were just trash. Then I saw it. Lying on the ground was a green, check-sized paper. It was my check. It must have fallen from my purse when I opened it up to get my car keys.

YELLOW STICKIES CAN HELP

"I put the grocery list on a wipe-off pad on the refrigerator. Every time I go to the supermarket, I write down the items on a post-it sticky note and put it in my coat pocket so it's there when I get to the store," says Judy, 39, mother of one son.

Was I lucky? Sure! Someone could have picked up that check and a bad person could have forged my name and cashed it. Or it could have been lost forever. But if I had not retraced my steps, I would have missed a valuable opportunity.

Of course, I only went to one place, and you may have been to five or six places since you knew you had the item. Start with the very first place you went to and look around. Then go to the next, and the next, and so on.

When You Have a Problem with Losing Keys

Many moms with ADD have the problem of losing their keys. Lost house keys, lost car keys, lost any other kind of keys that exist. Keys are small, easy to lose, and can be very hard to find. Here are some ideas to try:

- Keep an alternate set of keys. Or keep several sets, one at home, one at work.
- Keep your keys on a key ring. Bulky key rings are harder to lose than single keys.
- Keep the keys in the same place. Consider a key ring by the door. When you come in, the first thing you must do is place the keys on that key ring. You may not answer the telephone, get a drink, or do anything until you have done this.
- Think about getting a key finder. This is a device that you attach to your key ring. If you lose your keys (and they're within range), just whistle for your keys.
- You can also purchase a fancier key finder that has two parts. One is a device that you anchor to a stationary place, like next to your telephone. The other connects to your key chain. If you lose your keys, you activate the key finder (the anchored-down part) and it causes the key chain to beep.
- Consider camouflage. There are items that look like rocks but are really hollowed out, and you can hide an extra key in them. This is better than under the mat!
- If you trust your neighbor, give him or her an extra set.

Here are some ideas for keeping track of your car keys:

- Key finders work for them too.
- Buy a car that locks only from the outside. That way, you can't lock your keys in.
- Buy a device to hide an extra key that magnetically attaches at the wheel well.

Remembering: Part of Organizing

"I have good intentions but a lot of trouble following through with my great ideas," said Jill, 38, mother of two girls. "I have never been able to participate regularly with efforts like scouting because I forget about the meetings, and having two daughters with ADHD hasn't helped matters.

"I am a dynamo at the office but just cannot be relied upon at home. I missed my son's middle school graduation because I was out of town and had no idea until my oldest daughter called to scold me. It isn't that I don't care or don't want to do these things. It's like when I was a kid and couldn't remember to feed the dogs. I didn't want to kill them. I simply could not remember."

Assuming Jill would really like to be involved with scouting, is there anything she can do? Yes! There are many types of reminder devices, discussed later in this chapter, from whiteboards to calendars to computerized organizers, watches, and more.

Of course, Jill also needs to be careful that she is not taking on too many tasks, a common mistake that many women with ADD make. It's what I call the "saying-yes-too-much Problem."

▶ SAYING YES TOO MUCH

If you're like most mothers with ADD, you say yes far too often to many different requests, whether they're assignments at work, projects for your family, or jobs outside the family. I was a little dizzied by the numerous tasks my interviewees described taking on. But then, some people might be rattled by the workload I frequently place upon myself.

CUT BACK ON SURFACE AREAS

If you find that every spare surface in your home is covered with stuff, one tactic is to limit the number of surfaces. Cut back on coffee tables or end tables you don't really need and that are piled with newspapers and other debris.

What's So Hard about Saying No?

Why do we ADD moms say yes too much? Here's what I think are the primary components of saying yes to too many tasks: guilt, impulsiveness, curiosity, and time orientation.

1. **Guilt.** The Big "G" stands for major guilt and unfortunately, it's an impetus for the decisions of many moms with ADD. They can become so overwhelmed with guilt, and they are afraid to say no. This issue may also stem from a self-esteem problem; sometimes it's hard to separate how much is guilt and how much is low self-esteem.

DON'T BE AFRAID OF THE "N" WORD!

Many moms with ADD overburden themselves because they can't say the "N" word: No. They think it's bad to say no. They may drive the asker insane by giving 29 reasons why they can't do the job—but never actually use the N word. If you have a problem saying no, you have lots of company. However, it's still *you* who has to explain at the last minute why you can't do something you *promised* you would do.

A better tactic is to say no to all or most things that are beyond your time horizon—what you can see as "real." To know what your time horizon is, think of a difficult job and whether you could do it in a week. Then think of that same difficult job. Could you do it in six months? Three months? A month? A week?

Think about what timeframe would make the job seem not so bad for you. That is probably beyond your time horizon. Many readers may say, well of course, I could do that job in three months (six months, whatever), because that would give me *plenty* of time! But the reality is that most ADDers, no matter how hard they try, have a very strong tendency to put off things too long. If you are like that, and you can't do a hard job in two weeks now, you won't be able to do the hard job six months from now—in the two weeks you'll give yourself.

So identify your own personal time horizon, and learn to just say no when you really should use the N word.

Guilt-stricken mothers frequently agree to do jobs that they probably won't have time to handle. Or, if they take these tasks on, then they'd have to give up a few important things—like eating and sleeping—to make sure the jobs are done. I cover the issue of guilt and other difficult emotions felt by many —and offer some ideas on what to do about these disturbing feelings—in "Coping with Emotions" (Chapter Eleven).

2. **Impulsive yeses.** If you have to decide something fast, it's often easier to say yes than to say no, especially if you're an impulsive mom with ADD. And you want people to be happy and like you. Saying yes seems like the "right" answer. Remember this: The great Napoleon said that when you are surprised, it's best to say no first. It's easier to think it over and decide to say yes—than it is to retrieve the cavalry from a full charge!

USE YOUR CREATIVITY TO SOLVE ORGANIZING PROBLEMS

"If it makes sense for you, put kitchen towels and soaps in the kitchen cabinet. Use your address book for project ideas, your refrigerator for keeping nail polish, your ice bucket as a vase, and your ice cube trays as drawer organizers."

—Sheree Bykofsky in *500 Terrific Ideas for Organizing Everything* (Galahad Books, 1992)

---

3. **Curiouser and curiouser!** Most ADD moms are very intelligent and curious people with numerous interests. Often they agree to take on too many jobs because all of these tasks sound quite interesting. It can be hard to prioritize when you have ADD, so heck, let's do it all. Then later on when you get bogged down and are late, you must tell your child you really can't make all the food for the school picnic (as you promised), or you must tell your boss that the important project is going to be a few weeks late (although you had assured her that, this time, it would be there right on schedule). You may have to decide whom you will disappoint: your boss or your child.

Another problem is that when you break such promises, you'll find it lowers your self-esteem and can perpetuate a vicious circle. Break out! Learn to say no.

4. **Time disconnect.** For many moms with ADD, time is either *now* or *later.* As mentioned earlier, if a job doesn't have to be done until later, then it may seem like eons away. So why not say yes? It's not even a blip on your radar screen now.

Do You Have a Saying-Yes-Too-Much Problem?

You probably know if you have a saying-yes-too-much problem. But perhaps you don't. Or, if you do know, you may not realize where the problem lies. Some people overachieve with their family or at work or elsewhere. So where are you? Take my easy quiz to find out! Respond "yes" if the item sounds like you and "no" if it does not.

The Saying-Yes-Too-Much Self-Quiz	Yes	No
1. Your boss is excited about a new client and he asks for volunteers to work on this job. He looks at you. Do you volunteer?		
2. Your mom needs someone to plan the family reunion for a year from now. She asks you to organize the whole thing. Do you agree?		
3. Your son is failing in school. He tells you he needs home schooling. You have a job and know nothing about home schooling. You also hate this idea. Do you agree to home-school your child?		
4. Your aging father asks you to figure out all his finances for him. You work full time and have three children. What do you say to your father?		
5. Your clergyperson says it's time for the big festival. You've worked on it before, but now you are working overtime on a big project. What do you say?		
6. The hospital calls and asks you to volunteer. You've volunteered before, but you are really stressed out. But it's the hospital—the people who saved your father's life. They need to know now. What is your answer?		
7. Your daughter is active in Girl Scouts and also takes piano lessons. She is excited today because she has decided to be a library volunteer, and she signed up for Thursday nights. You will need to drive her there. Thursday is the one night you give yourself "off" from commitments. What do you say?		

If you find that taking this quiz reveals that you're inclined to do five or more of the previous items, you are probably overcommitting. Try this: When anyone asks you to perform *any* task that is due after today and that requires more than five minutes, either say "no" *or* hold yourself back from saying "yes." Instead, say that you must think about it. Resist the intense pressure that can sometimes emanate from others, who say that you've "always" done this before, that it's easy, it won't take much time, and so forth. No matter what, tell the person you must think about it and let them know.

This gives you time to actually consider the task and decide whether you want to—or can—do it. If you find that you do want to do it, and you have the time, energy, and resources, then contact the person in a day or so and tell him or her you'd be delighted to sign up for the job.

If you find that upon reflection, you really don't want to do it, or you don't have the time, energy, or resources (or all of the above), call the person back and politely decline. Do not offer excuse after excuse, and don't expect absolution. Just tell them that you can't do it this time and they'll need to get someone else. And be tough!

▶ TIME: IT ISN'T THAT FLEXIBLE EXCEPT ON STAR TREK

He lives as if his actions had no implications for the future, no effects on future needs, relationships or responsibilities. The short-term goal is invariably chosen over the long-term, with the exception of activities or projects capable of arousing the sluggish motivation-reward nexus in the brain. The present impulse dominates. It has been aptly said that people with ADD forget to remember the future.
—Gabor Mate, M.D., in *Scattered: How Attention Deficit Disorder Originates and What You Can Do About It* (Dutton, 1999)

Let's move further along the time-space continuum of problems related to ADD and into the problem of managing time. Many moms with ADD have a serious problem with being on time, meeting deadlines, and doing other time-related tasks. People talk about "time-saving" devices and not having enough time, or even about time speeding up or slowing down. But time doesn't do that! Time is a constant. It is our *perception* of time that makes it appear to drag on sometimes, and at other times seem to move like a rocket.

TIMERS CAN HELP WITH TIME PROBLEMS

"Using timers to complete tasks has been very helpful to me and my family," says Suzanne, 42, mother of two. "We set the timers to work on projects for specific times varying from 15 to 60 minutes. That usually makes it much easier to get things done." Arlene, mother of two, says if one session isn't enough to complete a task, then taking a break, or getting a snack (or a hug) makes it easier to continue. "I own about five kitchen timers that are scattered about the house."

This is important to understand and accept if you're an ADD mom, because most of us are involved in many different activities and are often rushing about madly. At some points in my children's life, I had to remind myself, "Okay, I am now going to pick up Jane at school from Brownies and bring her home and then go pick up Brian from Jimmy's house and then . . ." You can be doing so many different things that you confuse yourself. To paraphrase Thoreau, we need to "simply, simplify, our commitments."

When Time Becomes a Problem

The mom with ADD may be more likely to delay or procrastinate doing things that need to be done, such as boring bill paying, going to the dentist, and all those nonfun things that few of us like to think about. When you don't go to the dentist or doctor regularly, that's not good —you need to take care of yourself.

Many tasks, like having teeth or eyes checked, don't have to be done every month. So what do you have to do? The dreaded "S" word for many: scheduling.

AN EMERGENCY EVERYTHING BAG

"I have what I call my 'man overboard' bag with everything I could possibly need—wallet, cell phone, Filofax, book, umbrella, cosmetics, toothbrush, hairbrush, etc. (And, hopefully, my car keys.) I tote this bag everywhere, up, down, in, out, even to bed where I plunk it next to me on the floor. Without it, I'm truly lost," says Anne, 41, mother of two sons.

One tactic offered by author and psychologist Kathleen Nadeau for ADDers who have a tendency to put off work they've committed to is this: Write down on your calendar the date a project is due. Then go backward in your calendar and write down on different dates when various phases of the project must be done. For example, maybe the big carnival will be on May 15th. What are the tasks involved in planning?

Maybe you will need to order equipment or stock for the booths, sign up volunteers to work the booths, advertise the carnival in the local newspapers, or complete many other tasks. First write down the tasks, then go backward and figure out when is the last feasible date this task *must* be accomplished. And be realistic: Allow yourself some "wiggle room" of a few weeks or at least a few days.

MULTIPLE CALENDARS WORK FOR SOME MOMS WITH ADD

"I have calendars in nearly every room, just to keep track of the passage of time from month to month. The kitchen calendar is the family calendar and if the kids have an activity that isn't reported to me and isn't written on the kitchen calendar, then it doesn't exist and I won't be held responsible if it is forgotten," said Bev, 32, mother of two.

Author's Note: Multiple calendars may work for you too, but make sure you have a central calendar for *everything*.

This week, if your planning horizon really can't extend further, remember this acronym: KISS. It stands for "Keep It Simple, Silly."

Consider the Unchangeables

There are some immutable schedules of others that you will need to work within. For example, if your child starts school at 8:00 A.M., she must be there by 8. If she is late, she will be marked tardy. If she is frequently late, the school may levy punishment, or it could even affect her grade in some cases.

▶ MOM, ARE YOU ZONING OUT AGAIN? LEARNING TO LISTEN

"What on Earth are you thinking about so intensely? You look so serious!" Jim said to Jill. She was startled and said, "Oh nothing." And she really meant it. She had been staring off into space, but she wasn't really worried about anything. Nor did she even see what she was staring at. Her distractibility and inattentiveness were getting in the way.

Catch Yourself Clicking Off

How can you "catch" yourself clicking toward or in the off position? One way is with watches or timers, as many women suggest. Set timers or watches to go off at different times that are important.

Another possible solution is to use a watch, computer program, or some other device—perhaps a very loudly bonging grandfather clock—that will make noise every half-hour or every hour. I set my watch to beep every hour. Every so often, when I hear the loud beep, I actually do catch myself in the middle of daydreaming about nothing.

Lest anyone have the impression here that I am condemning daydreaming, I must add that I don't think there's anything inherently wrong with daydreaming. Often such daydreams are fun or stress-relieving, or they may lead to very creative ideas. Like when you're in the shower or deciding to lie down for a quick nap—often, unique thoughts may pop into your head. Many of my writing ideas come to me unbidden at such times.

Learning to Listen

An enormous number of problems have evolved because people didn't listen to each other, whether it was a cable warning about the imminent attack on Pearl Harbor, launching World War II or, on a far smaller scale, when your daughter thought you said you'd be at the mall to pick her up at six but you really said you'd be there at five.

Listening can be very difficult for the mom with ADD because of her inherent distractibility; however, most of us can learn the basics of good listening. Knowing these helpful tips may well give you the upper hand, or at least level the playing field with your non-ADD counterparts.

One problem with communication is the common tendency of most people to think about what *they* are going to say next and ignore what the other person is saying now. You're not necessarily being rude or trying to be inattentive. But most people think much faster than another person can speak. It's easy to fall into the trap of believing you can readily pick up the thread of what's going on in the conversation whenever you feel like jumping in again. Imagine yourself driving along a highway and daydreaming a bit because traffic is thin, the road is straight, and the weather is good. You know where you're going, but you miss your exit because you were not paying attention.

A conversation can be like that. You are talking with someone and then fade out to your own thoughts about what to eat for lunch or how to solve some problem. Just before you tuned out, the other person was talking about one topic. By the time you refocus, she's on an entirely new subject. You missed your listening "exit."

Here are some steps to get you started on the road to effective listening:

1. **Make a checklist.** If you are going to meet someone whom you know it's important to listen to, it's a good idea to prepare. Ask yourself:

- What is the primary reason I want to talk with this person?
- What information do I have that the other person may need?
- What do I expect or want this person to do?
- What am I willing to do?
- Are there specific, special needs or problems that are important to discuss?
- How much time will I probably have?

Maybe you have an appointment to see your child's teacher. You know *why* you are going to see him: because of Johnny's bad grades. But write down one or two sentences on what you expect from the encounter. Then ask yourself if these goals are realistically within reach of a good teacher.

For example, do you expect the teacher to transform Johnny from a child receiving failing grades into a straight-A student? Teachers rarely can help your child achieve that goal for you, as wonderful as it sounds. Or, do you want improved grades, preferably passing ones? That is a more likely goal to work toward.

Next, whether you realize it or not, you have a lot of information to provide in a face-to-face interchange. Before your meeting, write down key points you want to get across, such as what you feel are the primary problems, how severe they are, and of course, what you hope the teacher or other person will do for you.

It is easy to forget information you wanted to address (especially if you are naturally distractible). Your checklist can avoid this problem.

2. **Bring documentation.** Another step in preparing for effective communication is to bring helpful items. For example, if Susie has received rave reviews for her artwork, bring some samples if it might help. The new teacher may have no idea of Susie's artistic talent, and it could be a way to reach her. If you or your child just had x-rays or lab tests and you are seeing a new doctor, bring those results with you! You may not need those tests repeated, and they can provide important information.

3. **Talk about what's bothering you.** If the other person doesn't broach the subject that concerns *you* most, you should bring it up. In fact, don't wait too long to do so. Give the person an opportunity to greet you and make at least one comment before you leap into your area of distress. But don't wait until it's time to leave and then do a sudden "Oh, by the way," and drop a bombshell. That strategy won't work well, and it's really annoying.

4. **Take notes.** It's a good idea to take simple notes and review them with the person you're talking with. For example, if she provides instructions or important information, jot it down. Try to summarize her main points. Then at the end, say, "Ms. Brown, I think the most important things you want me to do are . . ." If you're mistaken, she'll correct you; and then you'll know what's expected.

5. **Ask questions.** Often we don't understand what the other person is trying to communicate—for a variety of reasons. For example, she may be using "slanguage" (I made that up)—words or phrases understandable to some groups but not others. If she uses terminology you don't understand, ask what it means. If she begins to rattle off numbers and they are meaningless to you, ask if this means that things are better or worse than before.

Your child's coach may have known someone with a similar problem who found a workable solution, a solution that might be effective in your child's case too. Provide information that may help you both collaborate to come up with a good plan.

Many parents worry about asking questions or requesting clarification. They fear if they ask something, the other person will think they are not smart. Be aware that most people don't expect you to know as much about their field of expertise as they know. And they would usually prefer you to ask questions while you're there. This is much better than calling back later, trying to relay messages through an assistant.

6. **Collaborate in decision-making.** When the person you are speaking with feels he has enough information, he'll make recommendations. Consider each recommendation seriously and respond. Let's say your conference is with a teacher. Tell her if you can't comply with a request. For example, if a teacher wants you to spend three hours a night helping your child with homework, this may be impos-

sible for a tired mom with ADD who can barely focus on eating her dinner, let alone slogging through homework with a frustrated child.

Do you understand what the teacher is advising you to do? If so, say so. If you don't understand certain terms or are confused by what she is recommending, get clarification. How? One good way is to summarize what you think she has said, and ask her if this is right. "I think you are telling me I should have Susie work on her homework within an hour after she comes home for at least a week and see if that improves her ability to finish her work on time. Is that right?" If it isn't correct, the teacher will tell you what he really meant.

▶ BLURTING OUT COMMENTS: GETTING A GRIP ON THAT TONGUE

As I mentioned earlier, one problem many of us have is saying what we mean—a little bit too much. I mean, what we *really* mean or sometimes what we're really thinking and it doesn't come out quite right. Our inner censor is bypassed. Often it would be better to say little or nothing —or maybe murmur some positive comment.

"I have often been accused of not thinking before talking. That's not even half-true. I often talked *while* I was thinking," said Gail, 37, and a mother of two. Her brain and her mouth seem to operate simultaneously. She has trouble with the "inhibition" part, the aspect of the brain that enables a person to process a thought before spewing it out.

Let me give you an example of one of *my* embarrassing moments. I was single, not a mother yet, and was an Air Force lieutenant—probably a very different situation from many readers, but this incident illustrates my point. I had just arrived at a Saturday morning picnic and of course everyone, including me, was wearing "civilian" clothes rather than our uniforms. I was standing among a large group of people when someone came over to me and said loudly, "Hey! How come you didn't say hi to me, Lieutenant?"

I realized he was a sergeant who worked for me, but he looked different out of uniform. I said, "I'm sorry! I didn't recognize you with clothes on!"

As you can imagine, that was a major "oops." When I realized what I had said, versus what I meant ("you look really different out of uniform"), my face blazed bright red, to the great hilarity of all. The poor man was as embarrassed as I was, but he forgave me. I didn't know I had ADD then—and wish that I had known!

That particular incident entertained people, but it doesn't always amuse others when we blurt out thoughts. Sometimes we can get into pretty hot water with friends, coworkers, and family members when words pour out, unthinkingly.

Here's where you can enlist the help of others in your family and/or at work if you have a serious blurting-out problem. Tell the person who you'd like to help you that you know you sometimes blurt out comments before thinking. Also add that you realize others can't anticipate your thoughts to "save" you each time from disaster. But ask her, if she notices you starting to say something when it would be better to be quiet, to signal you.

One signal could be for the person to hold up the hands with fingers out, to illustrate, "take ten." Another signal could be similar to those used by referees in football to signal a time-out.

There are innumerable kinds of signals that you and she can consider using as "blurt attack pending" reminders. Just remember to make it simple: Use only one kind of signal so you'll know exactly what she means—instead of wondering if maybe she's having a nervous breakdown.

Another tactic is recommended by Kathleen Nadeau in her book, *ADD in the Workplace: Choices, Changes, and Challenges* (Brunner/Mazel, 1997). To prevent yourself from blurting out remarks at meetings, train yourself to take notes and write down your comments before you say them. Often people with ADD blurt out comments because they're afraid if they don't say what's on their minds right *now*, that thought will disappear and be lost forever in the Bermuda Triangle of their brains.

This strategy of writing things down can serve several purposes. First, it relieves you of the fear of losing that thought. Second, if you write it down and then read it, you're more likely to see if it's a comment that could be considered tactless— and you won't say it. The notes will also help remind you of what was said at a meeting. Taking notes can also remind you that you are *at* a meeting and help keep you on task.

▶ HYPERREACTIVITY TO STIMULI

My son talks all the time and is a constant barrage of noise. It's extremely hard for a parent with no ability to screen out stimuli and it exacerbates my ADD meltdown. I am constantly asking him to please stop talking before I drive off the road, microwave the cat, pour juice on my cereal, etc.
—Judy, 39, mother of one son

Some people with ADD are highly reactive to certain stimuli. They may not be able to tolerate loud sounds; or they may have difficulty in shopping malls, especially at Christmas, because of so many people, so many things.

No Spicy Clothes

Some people with ADD are hyperreactive to touch or to things that touch them. For example, Lily, 45, says her son was always sensitive to certain clothes from infancy. The only clothes that seemed to make him comfortable were 100 percent cotton.

If Lily put a cotton and polyester shirt on Tommy, her toddler could tell right away that it didn't feel right. He usually told Lily the shirt was "wrong" or "too spicy"—presumably transposing the use of the word from overly spiced food he didn't like.

Although Lily did buy Tommy 100 percent cotton clothes, she thought it was an affectation or quirk. That is, until one day when she caught herself in a department store, in the act of feeling clothes to see if they "felt right." She'd just selected a beautiful dress that would be perfect for a party she'd be going to; but when she ran her hands over it, it felt harsh and rough and she knew she couldn't wear it.

Lily began wondering if some clothes were "spicy" to her. She realized that ever since she could remember, one of her main criteria in choosing clothes was, did they *feel* right? If not, she wouldn't buy them. Or, if she did, she'd wear the item once—or never. She realized Tommy felt the same way that she did.

Adaptations to Hyperreactivity

If you are hyperreactive to some stimuli, you may be able to accommodate the problem if it can't be ignored. You may be able to change your work environment as well. If necessary, you can cite the Americans with Disabilities Act as a reason for your employer to provide accommodations, such as white-noise machines and other devices or actions that can be taken in the workplace. Read "Juggling Family and Work: The Workplace" (Chapter Five) for more information.

Here is a chart of possible actions to take if you are hypersensitive to stimuli.

Problem	Possible Solutions
Hypersensitive to loud sounds	Wear headphones or ear plugs to block outside noise. Turn down the phone ringer, or screen calls with Caller ID or answering machine. Turn the TV off and read the captions.
Hypersensitive to touch	Wear comfortable clothes—don't be a "fashion slave." Wear natural fabrics like cotton. Wear no makeup or hypoallergenic makeup. Choose mild detergents
Hypersensitive to crowds	Avoid crowds. Shop in off-hours (early or late). Use headphones. If crowds can't be avoided, take privacy breaks.

▶ HIGH- AND LOW-TECH SOLUTIONS CAN HELP

There are good solutions available that can help you with ADD-related problems, whether they are space, time or distractability problems or hyperreactivity problems. Some solutions are high-tech and some are distinctly "low-tech," such as calendars.

Low-Tech Solutions

I must make a to-do list every day or I will forget what to do!
—Laurie, 31, mother of two boys

You don't have to be a computer genius or lover of the latest gadget to benefit from devices to help you resolve the problems ADD can bring. Often very low-tech and everyday items you probably take for granted can help—such as calendars or lists.

1. **Calendars.** Many women with ADD could not function without their calendars. It's where we write down important appointments as well as give ourselves reminders to buy birthday or holiday gifts. Many also use their calendars to jot down important phone numbers, such as your child's school, the pediatrician's number, and so forth. I prefer a spiral-bound calendar with a page for each day, but others prefer a wall-sized monthly calendar that they hang up.

"I am lost without my datebook and calendar," says Jean, 32, mom of three children. "I don't care how many appointment cards I get—they all get lost really fast!"

Elaine, 29, mother of one, says she relies on her whiteboard in the kitchen. "It's our message center for phone messages, shopping lists, weekly activities, and menus."

2. **Appointment boards.** "I use a huge dry-erase board in my kitchen. It's been a life saver for me because now I have appointments and important to-do things in one place!" says Emma, 29, mother of one.

3. **Daytimers/planners.** Many mothers rely on dayplanners, which include not only a calendar but also an address book and a place to keep notes. Those who rely on their dayplanners swear they could not possibly function without them. There are a broad variety of dayplanners, from popularly known and pricey brands to the inexpensive kind you can buy at K-Mart.

CLIP IMPORTANT ITEMS TOGETHER

I use a copyholder to keep track of urgent bills, papers, prescriptions, etc. This is a plastic clipboard slightly larger than 81/2" X 11" with a clip on top. It's connected to a flexible arm attached to my desk. I can cram about 20 papers under the clip. It is next to my computer, and I can't *not* see it. I can't lose it—it's connected to my desk!

High-Tech Devices

You may also wish to take advantage of the high-tech devices that can help you resolve an array of ADD-related problems. Many people swear by their pagers and computers and say they would be lost without them.

1. **Pagers.** A pager is a much more common device than in past years; in fact, some parents give them to schoolchildren so they can page their children if they're late in getting home from a date! Some businesses give their employees pagers. Other people get their own pagers and pay $20–$30 a month (or more, if paged very frequently). Another good feature of a pager is if you lose it nearby, you can call yourself and hear the pager go off.

Some women use the alarm feature of their pagers. "If my pager didn't go off at 5:30, I'd never remember to take my medicine!" said Laurie.

If you are hypersensitive to sounds and the beep of a pager would make you visibly leap, you might be better off with a pager that pulsates instead. The throbbing of the pager can make a low drone, but it primarily uses a persistent pulsation to attract its owner's attention.

2. **Computer organizers or programs.** Several mothers told me they relied on their Palm Pilot computer organizers. "It's my brain! I could not function without it," emphasized Jessie, 35, mother of three children ages, 5, 8, and 10.

A TEACHER'S PLANNING CALENDAR CAN HELP NON-TEACHERS TOO

I love the teacher's planning calendar I use for myself. I need to see the big picture. You can open it up and see an entire month, with big boxes to write in.

—Joyce, 32, mother of three

Added Roberta, 39 and parent to one daughter, "I only write in the Palm Pilot that automatically downloads information into the datebook and notes on the computer so I won't mess up the information."

Kathy, 41, mother of two girls, says, "At work I use the calendar on the computer and it has a reminder system. I set it to remind me of appointments, thirty minutes beforehand. Sometimes I set it to remind me to *stop* working and clear up, a half hour before it was time to get off work!"

Another mom, Lucy, 36, mother of two children, says "I programmed a beep to ring on my computer every fifteen minutes to remind me of time passing. It breaks me out of that zombie-state I get into sometimes—some people call it being 'inattentive.' The ringing brings me back to reality fast!"

Of course, many men and women who do *not* have ADD find computer organizers helpful devices too. But for the mom with ADD who relies on her organizer, it's often much more than a helpful aid—it's a lifeline.

3. **Watches.** Even a "plain old" watch today can be an important device for a mom with ADD. Most watches include not only the time but also the date—and that is an easy thing to forget! Many watches also tell you what day it is, if you have a problem remembering whether it is Tuesday or Wednesday. That can be very helpful if you must perform some task every Wednesday; for example, pick up Cindy after band practice because she doesn't take the bus home that day.

There are also fancier watches that you can purchase that pulsate or beep, or both, every hour or only on certain times and dates. I use a watch, which also provides a visual reminder: The watch flashes bright blue off and on as it pulsates. Thus, I receive a sensory reminder and a visual reminder.

4. **Digital voice recorders.** If you don't like writing notes to yourself and you respond better to auditory (sound) stimuli, then consider using a digital voice recorder. This is a device with no tape in it, but it holds varying amounts of information. They sell for about $50 at Radio Shack and other retailers. Thus, you can turn it on at work or at home and tell yourself you need to be sure to do A, B, and C. Then, when you arrive at work or home, you can play back the recorder reminders to yourself.

ALTERNATIVES TO WHITE-NOISE MACHINES
- **Tune the TV to a channel with no station, and turn the volume up.**
- **Try a fan.**
- **If you own an air-cleaning machine, it can double as a sound masker.**

---

5. **White-noise generators.** Many find white-noise generators or "sound maskers" are important aids to blocking distractions. A white-noise generator makes a sound similar to, but not as annoying as, static on a television or radio. It can help many people block noises they would otherwise pay attention to rather than concentrating on a task they want to perform. White-noise generators come in all sizes, shapes, and prices. Some devices include other sounds, such as falling rain, the wind, the ocean, and so forth.

Some women with ADD state they really could not cope without their "noise machines." White-noise generators can cost from $100 to several hundred dollars or more. Make sure it's a device for personal use rather than industrial or laboratory use—those are much more expensive.

In this chapter, I covered solutions to help the mom with ADD counteract some key problems that attention deficit disorder can bring, such as disorganization, blurting out comments, losing items, and other problems.

4

Juggling Family and Work: The Family

"I'm just a sponge for whatever anyone needs or wants—and today I was completely wrung out," said Donna, 35. By the time she picked up her six-year-old son Chad at day care at 6:30, half an hour late, she had little energy or patience and wearily agreed to pay the fine for being late to arrive.

After they arrived home, Donna somehow managed to throw together dinner before her husband Jim arrived. After dinner and the dishes, she walked about picking up a week's worth of old newspapers and doing general cleanup. Donna actually surprised herself when Chad suddenly asked if she had signed the school permission slip yet, and she blew up at him, invoking tears on his part and instant remorse on hers. Then she rushed around contritely and frantically trying to find that permission slip—for over an hour. Which pile could it possibly be in?

Chad was really upset, not only because he'd been unfairly yelled at but also because he couldn't go on the trip without the form and the trip was tomorrow. Finally at nearly 11 P.M. and hours after a still-upset Chad had fallen asleep, Donna found the permission slip stuffed under one of the sofa cushions. Another day, another crisis. She wouldn't have thought it was possible to feel even more wrung out—but she did.

Is this a rare scenario? Partly yes and partly no; many women today feel overworked and overstressed. The difference is that Donna has ADD. For her, stress greatly exacerbates her symptoms of inattentiveness and confusion, making her life even more difficult. She can't make her ADD go away altogether, even though the medications help her. But there are actions Donna could take to make life easier on the home front.

If you're like Donna and feeling overwhelmed by everything that's going on at home, this chapter offers some ideas for organizing yourself on the homefront, including:

- An analysis of Donna's problems
- Creating a plan
- Working on skills for home
- Staying firm: not wimping out
- Working out solutions with family members
- Keeping boundaries in mind (yours and theirs)

▶ **ANALYZING DONNA**

Clearly, Donna is one stressed lady, and she was unable to get Chad out of day care on time. This may have happened to her before—probably has. Donna needs to find another solution. Maybe she needs different childcare—discussed in "Juggling Family and Work: The Workplace." (Chapter Five). Maybe she could ask her husband to pick up Chad.

Arriving home, Donna is the one to make dinner. Maybe husband Jim would have made dinner, even though he came home later. Or he could have brought home some takeout (as could Donna).

After dinner, Donna washed the dishes. Why not get a dishwasher? Or dump them in soapy water if you were exhausted as Donna was and Jim didn't want to do them either?

As for Chad's school permission form, Donna needs to create a system that works for her right away, because Chad is only 6 and the stream of paper coming home is only going to get bigger and bigger. This is an organization problem Donna needs to work on. Maybe she could stick it on the refrigerator with a magnet or tack it to the wall. Or, better yet, sign the thing as soon as Chad gives it to her and have him return it early.

BE CREATIVE AT PROBLEM-SOLVING ON THE HOMEFRONT

Here's some advice from James Thornton, author of *Chore Wars*:

"Women tend to communicate their request verbally—that is, if you want your partner to do something, you ask him to do it. If this fails, odds are you'll just ask again—but in a louder and angrier voice. This tends to make him feel you're trying to control him, and he becomes even less likely to do what you want. So instead of talking, try taking creative action. One example: for fifty years, one wife had pleaded with her husband not to come to the dinner table with his shirt off. For fifty years, he had ignored her requests . . . [One day] she decided to try taking off her own shirt at the dinner table. Her husband never ate shirtless again."

Source: James Thornton, author of *Chore Wars: How Households Can Share the Work and Keep the Peace* (Conari Press, Berkeley, California, 1997).

▶ **CREATE A PLAN**

In the previous chapter, I covered ideas and tools that can help you overcome problems with impulsivity, organization, impatience and other typical traits of many moms with ADD. But you also need a working plan. How do you develop one? First, define your own primary problems. Then consider the goals that you'd like to achieve and define strategies that can help you get there from here.

These are the basic steps:

1. Determine the primary problems.

2. Write down and analyze your goals in terms of your weaknesses and strengths.

3. Develop workable strategies.

4. Create systems to get things done, your way.

Determine the Primary Problems

You can't solve your main problems until you're clear on what they are. Even if you think you are quite certain that you know what your key problems are, do this exercise anyway. Get a piece of paper and a pen or pencil. Draw a line down the middle of the paper so that you now have two columns. Without thinking about it very much, jot down your top five or six problems in one of the columns. It doesn't matter if they are related to your ADD or not. Just make the list.

Take a look at what you've written and figure out what ADD category your problems fit closest. For example, you may blurt out what's on your mind and upset people. That's an impulsivity issue. Or let's say you lose many items, and your husband thinks you'd lose your head if it weren't connected to your body. That's organization. Write down the category of each problem in the other column. Some ADD characteristics to consider could be disorganization, distractibility, procrastination, losing things, forgetting, saying yes when you should have said no, hyperactivity, and inattentiveness. Your list may look like this when you're done:

Problem	Category of Problem
People are always mad at me for being late.	Disorganization; possibly "zoning out"
I lose everything! I should get a job losing things; I could go far because I'm so good at it!	Organization/distractibility
I say things that I shouldn't because I speak and *then* think.	Impulsivity
I can't seem to sit still.	Hyperactivity

I have a terrible cold that won't go away.	Not ADD
I think my husband is going to divorce me.	
He says I don't listen and must not care about him.	inattentiveness
My neighbor is mad at me because I told our other neighbor something she told me in confidence. It just slipped out!	Impulsivity

After you've made your list, rank the problems from 1 for most important to the highest number for least important.

Once you've worked on identifying which aspects of ADD are most troublesome to you, then you can begin work on resolving them, starting with the worst and working your way down. Maybe you thought hyperactivity was your worst problem, but you now see that disorganization is really bogging you down. Organization problems are covered in, "Working on Solutions to Common ADD Problems" (Chapter Three). Go back and see if you can find some solutions that would work for you there.

The point is, it's important to identify the root element of what is really bothering you. Once you know what it is, then you can work to improve that situation or problem. We moms with ADD are very creative people, and we don't give up easily either. You can be relentless at working to resolve the issues that cause you the most distress.

Write Down Your Goals

**When I'm at work, home doesn't exist for me, so I forget to make appointments or to remember things I need to take care of on breaks or at the end of the day.
When I'm at home, work ceases to exist and I forget to do work I need to do, planning, and phone calls.**
—Carol, mother of one child

In addition to identifying your problems, it's also good to determine your primary goals. Maybe your problems aren't really as detrimental to your goals as you think.

Create another chart with two columns, like the following one Tracey made. In one column, write down areas where you'd like to improve. In the other column, write down things you do well now. You can't leave this column blank! Write down something. I am a strong believer that by thinking about your weak points *and* your strong points, often you can come up with a creative solution to a problem.

Let's look at Tracey's list.

Things I Want to Do Better	Things I Do Well Now
Be more patient.	I'm good with animals.
Be more punctual.	I love to read.
Get in better shape.	I love music.

Develop Workable Strategies

Can you see any possible patterns or solutions here? I can! Tracey thinks she is too impatient. She also loves animals. Odds are, she's probably fairly patient with puppies, kittens, bunnies, or other animals. Maybe the next time she is feeling impatient, Tracy could think of a big white rabbit with a twitching nose. Sounds silly, but it might just calm her down!

Okay, punctuality is another problem she identified. Tracey loves to read. She could reward herself with one hour of reading time if she is on time to an appointment. This is a positive reinforcement and based on Tracey's personal frame of reference.

Tracey also wants to get into better shape. She's a music lover. This is easy, falling off a log! Tracey should wear her Walkman while she's jogging or doing housework or whatever active exercise will help get her into shape.

You don't have to solve one problem with whatever you wrote next to it on the page. For example, impatient Tracey could calm herself down by playing music. Animal-loving Tracey could get herself in shape by taking the dog for long walks. Moms with ADD can use their innate creativity to come up with many good solutions.

Create Systems to Get Things Done, Your Way

Many people seem to think there's only one right way and one wrong way to do everything. The reality is that, although some things can be done only one way, most goals can be arrived at in a variety of ways. What you need to do is come up with ideas on what will particularly motivate you to achieve your goals, whether it's small rewards to yourself, the thrill of imagining yourself completing the task, or some other method that gets you from point A to point B.

Most people may travel in a straight line from A to B, but maybe you'd rather go to C, D, and E before heading toward B—a pattern common to many women with ADD. Will the end result be the same, or just as good? It might be.

▶ SKILLS TO WORK ON AT HOME

Often you can use skills that you have developed on the job to use at home. Two primary skills many moms need to work on are patience and firmness. Let's begin with a look at patience; firmness is addressed in the next section.

Patience Can Be a Virtue: Working on It

Because of a tendency of many moms with ADD to live in the "now," sometimes we can be impatient with others more ponderous in their thoughts and actions. In addition, sometimes we become impatient at *things*—like machines or traffic lights—that are too slow for us. We may even utter nasty comments to these inanimate objects. In the meantime, as we are impatient and veering sharply toward anger, we may be raising our own blood pressure.

How Impatient Are You? Take This Self-Test!

Put a check mark or an *X* next to the statements that are true in your case.

❑ 1. When I am stopped in traffic at a red light, I feel like it is never going to change.

❑ 2. If I am waiting to see my doctor and have waited more than fifteen minutes, I think that's long enough and tell the staff so.

❑ 3. Those "voice mail" phone systems that tell you to dial 1 if this, 2 if that, or 3 or 10 really drive me crazy! If I reach one, my first impulse is to hang up.

❑ 4. I tell my computer to "hurry up" when logging on to my Internet provider or going to a website.

❑ 5. I'll change lines at the checkout counter at the supermarket three or four times to get to a faster-moving line.

❑ 6. When I'm listening to someone, I want him or her to *get to the point*. No small talk for me.

❑ 7. If the speed limit is 45 and I'm behind a person going 30, it makes me totally nuts.

❑ 8. If someone wants to take a scenic route, 100 miles out of the way, I object! We should go on the interstate highway, it's faster.

❑ 9. I get impatient at fast-food restaurants. Service is too slow!

If you made four or more check marks, you probably have a patience problem.

Develop Tactics and Strategies to Ratchet Up Your Patience Quotient

You can use meditation, relaxation therapy, yoga, or any number of ways to increase your patience quotient. Another way to slow down is to ask these questions:

- Is it essential that this be done right now?
- If this is done slower, could it be done better?
- Is this really worth worrying about?

Be Firm: Sometimes Moms with ADD "Wimp Out"

You have a rule that on school nights, your daughter must be in bed by 10 P.M. But tonight she says she wants to watch a "special show" on television. You're really exhausted from working hard all day, and the last thing you feel like doing is arguing. Besides, she's been really good lately.

Are You Giving in Too Much?

It's okay to give in once in awhile to your children's requests that run contrary to the rules. But if you find yourself giving in as frequently as daily, or even several times a week, then you are not being consistent in following your own rules. You may also find that you are teaching your children the following lessons:

- If you scream, cry, or beg long and loud enough, Mom will give in.
- If you behave well for a day or two, you can have whatever you want.
- The rules don't really matter.

We moms with ADD are flexible and spontaneous people. But we also need to remember that children need some structure. Do some self-examination. Pay attention to how often you are giving in on rules you've set.

If you find that you have been too loose on the rules, don't overcorrect and veer off into becoming a monster dictator. Instead, try to make subtle but firm course corrections until you're where you want yourself and your children to be. Also, expect a lot of testing. Children like getting their way. If you decide you're going to enforce the rules, expect some negative feedback. Keep your cool and hold fast to your position.

Rulemaking vs. Chaos: You Can Find a Balance

Sometimes when adults with ADD hear words like *rules,* they tend to clutch up and think, "Oh, no, not that! Anything but that!" It's not that we are rebellious nonconformists, although some of us are. Instead, the problem is that it's hard enough to follow the rules that we are supposed to be complying with *now.* So how can we possibly cope with even *more* rules?

The good news is that if *you* are the rulemaker (in collaboration with your spouse and other family members—you need their buy-in!) then you have some control over the rules. You can design them and figure out how to follow them. You can't make the rules at your job (unless you're the owner of the company), and often you can't make rules regarding your children's activities or schooling. But you *can* create order out of some of the chaos in your life by creating some operational rules for yourself.

You decide which rules are important, and which rules cannot and must not be broken except under very special circumstances—to be defined by you.

▶ WORKING OUT SOLUTIONS WITH FAMILY MEMBERS

It's very important for the mom with ADD to obtain cooperation from family members. You should not do all this stuff on your own! If you try to do it solo, you will become frustrated, resentful, and anxious. So get the troops in on the plan with you.

Do *not* make the mistake of thinking you can do everything on your own, if only you "work hard enough." Please! Didn't you hear that enough as a child and get frustrated enough at others who said it to you? If you've forgotten, then remind yourself!

Working hard is not the only thing. You need to work with your other family members, my next topic on the agenda.

Having a Family Meeting

You need your other family members to "buy in" to a plan for achieving family goals such as housecleaning, planning vacations, and other tasks that affect you all. Sure, you are the Parent. But have you also heard of another capital P, as in "Passive resistance?" If your significant other or children are not really agreeing with your ideas, you'll encounter plenty of foot dragging. You need a plan that's both workable and one that family members will comply with.

The best idea is to have some sort of plan or ideas when you meet with your family. You should also allow other family members, even a three-year-old child, to comment on your ideas and offer suggestions. Little Tiffany may surprise you!

DON'T BE "IT" ALL THE TIME

Collaborate with your family on working out a family schedule for necessary household tasks, keeping in mind you should not allow yourself to become "It"—the one who does everything that must be done that others don't feel like doing.

It's not a democracy, because Mom (and Dad too, if you are married) gets to make final decisions for the family. But when children feel it's more of a benign dictatorship than total authoritarian rule and also feel you will at least consider their ideas, they are far more likely to cooperate.

Whatever rules you decide upon, make sure that everyone understands them. When they violate the rules—and they will—use gentle reminders. Don't be surprised if a child reminds *you* that you're breaking a rule. If that happens, take it with good humor and grace. Set a time when everyone in the family can be home. Choose a time that seems good to you, and tell each member about it. If no complaints are registered, write down the date and time and post it on the refrigerator or your whiteboard where everyone can easily see it. Caution: Don't make the time too far off into the future. Try to make it sometime this week.

Sample of Ten Possible Rules for Family Meeting (Adapt these rules to your family.)

1. Mom, Dad, or whoever called the meeting should have a plan for what needs to be discussed. It should be written down whenever possible.

2. After everyone is there, the person who called the meeting should explain what he or she wants to discuss and list any problem-solving ideas to be presented.

3. Family members should listen and not talk when someone else is speaking.

4. Family members should not interrupt the speaker; however, the person with the "floor" should not hog it. If others want to speak, give them a chance.

5. Everyone should be allowed to express an opinion, no matter how old or young.

6. When an opinion is expressed, it should not be laughed at or ridiculed—unless it was clearly a joke. Ideas that may sound silly can often be adapted into very good solutions.

7. If an idea does sound workable, discuss how to implement it.

8. The meeting should not last longer than an hour, unless *all* members want it to.

9. A meeting is not a failure if nothing gets accomplished. Ideas have still been planted, and they may need time to germinate.

10. A meeting is not a failure if someone gets annoyed with someone else. This could be a chance to air grievances that the rest of the family didn't know about.

Issues for the Family

Here are some issues that family members may work out at a family meeting.

- Chores: Who does what, and when.
- Mandatory rules for everyone: What are they? Example—last one in locks the front door.
- Primary responsibilities: Who is mostly responsible for feeding the cat or dog?
- In-fighting: How can bickering between family members be resolved?

▶ **DON'T FORGET BOUNDARIES! YOURS AND THEIRS**

Put some barbed-wire boundaries around your personal time, where and when you can regroup and recharge.
—ADD coach and author Kate Kelly

It's common for people with ADD not to notice the boundaries of others, or to allow their own boundaries to be "invaded." What is a boundary and why is it important?

Personal Boundaries

Most people think of a boundary as a geographical divider, such as the boundary between the United States and Canada. But there are also personal boundaries, such as how close you may stand next to a person—which also depends on whether that person is a total stranger to you, your child, or your lover. Social boundaries vary in different cultures. In some countries, it is not rude to be very close to a complete stranger.

There are also personal territorial boundaries, such as your home or your bedroom. Or your clothes and your purse—including who may use these items or even touch them. You may not mind if your husband looks in your purse for a ten-dollar bill. But you might mind it a lot if it's your child looking through your purse.

Another boundary could be time: your time for yourself versus an attempt by someone trying to monopolize your time. Or your husband's time for work and interests.

There could also be boundaries of feelings; you might wish to share your joy or grief with people close to you while not telling others how you feel, because it's *private*.

In general, we tacitly understand each other's boundaries; however, sometimes moms with ADD aren't so clear. That's when trouble can occur.

Violating Personal Boundaries

It's easy to make a boundary mistake when you are distractible, crisis-oriented, excitable, and so forth. In the heat of the moment, you can tread on the emotional toes of the people who mean the most to you.

YOUR INWARD VIEW OF YOU

Michigan therapist and author Sari Solden says it's very important for moms with ADD to realize that taking medication for a few weeks or months is often not enough—although it can help a lot.

Another problem: the underlying beliefs and negative thoughts that moms with ADD may have about themselves. Solden says some clients ask how they could make their kids be unlike them. Instead, she recommends that moms with ADD realize that they are in a unique position to show empathy and caring, especially if their children have ADD too.

She also says our children model themselves on us, and if we are always putting ourselves down, how can we wonder about why our kids have a poor self-image?

Solden advises moms with ADD to build on their strengths and abilities rather than constantly worry about what they're bad at.

So how do you avoid this problem? One way is to tell the people you care about that sometimes you say and do things without thinking, and please tell you if you have offended them. Another way is to look, really look, at the people you care about and observe their face and body language. Arms folded across the chest, a frown, a person staring at the floor—these are only a few signs of a person who is not happy. This doesn't necessarily mean you were the cause of this distress, or even that it's a boundary issue. But you should ask. Here are a few possible boundary violations:

- Telling your teenage son's girlfriend about cute things he did as an infant.
- Insisting on talking to your daughter while she's in the bathroom. A lot of people want to be left alone then!
- Forcing a hug on a cringing adolescent. Teenagers may not wish to be touched.
- Telling a visiting child that of course your child would be happy to "share" his favorite toy. Maybe he wouldn't be.
- Eating the food off your spouse's plate in a restaurant without asking. This drives some people really crazy.

In this chapter, I focused primarily on major homefront battles for the mom with ADD, such as creating a plan to resolve problems at home and working on important skills such as patience and understanding boundaries.

5

Juggling Family and Work: The Workplace

I have structured my life so that I work entirely alone and have the flexibility to accommodate my attention problems. It may take me twelve hours to accomplish three hours of work—but no one has to know it except me.
—Judy, 39, freelance writer and parent of one son

ADD affects us in our work life, too—which then has impacts on our family life, which then has impacts on our work life, and then back to our family life. This chapter is about getting it together at work, including resolving the following common challenges:

- Finding and evaluating good childcare
- Working at an ADD-friendly job
- Worrying about kids when you're at work—and about work when you're at home
- Knowing about laws that may help you in the workplace

▶ FINDING AND EVALUATING CHILDCARE

One key problem for many moms—with or without ADD—is that in order to work, you must make a plan for someone to care for your children. Even if you are able to work at home, most mothers must arrange for others to watch their small children for some period of time so they can do their work.

When a mom has ADD, her concomitant problems of forgetfulness and impulsivity can cause direct problems or give her trouble in resolving problems that occur as an indirect result. Many problems are solvable if you keep the points in the following sections in mind.

Choosing Childcare

When selecting a childcare facility, it's important to *resist* any natural tendency toward impulsive behavior or last-minute decisions. In fact, according to Ann Douglas, author of *The Unofficial Guide to Childcare* (IDG Books, 1999), the biggest mistake that parents make when choosing childcare is leaving their search to the absolute last possible minute. "I recommend that parents start looking at least three months before they know they'll be needing childcare," says Douglas.

LOCATION, LOCATION, LOCATION

If another person, such as your husband or significant other, will also pick up your child, consider both workplaces. If you work on opposite ends of the city, can you find a childcare center that's midway? Of course, the quality of the center should be your foremost concern.

Use your natural creativity as well as the inherent curiosity of most moms with ADD. Ask plenty of questions, and be sure to take a walk around every facility that you are considering. If you can hyperfocus, use that capacity: Hyperfocus on finding all potential childcare facilities and comparing and contrasting them.

Evaluating a Facility

Many of us ADD moms have a tendency to be impatient as well as impulsive. However, the childcare decision is such a major one that it's important to be very careful. Whenever possible, avoid rushing this choice.

Make a reasoned comparison between the available options, as a mother committed to her children's safety and welfare should be. Make sure you actually visit any facility you are considering for your child before you make a commitment to that facility. Take a long hard look at each center while you're there.

Good Facilities

To help you determine how good a childcare center is, look at the following factors (and do not limit your search to these aspects alone):

- *The caregiver/child ratio.* See the following chart on what the experts recommend.
- *General cleanliness of the childcare center.* Expect some messes, because children are running around everywhere. But the center should not reek of urine or feces and should look relatively clean.

- *The overall attitude of the staff.* Do they really like children?
- *Do you see any problems with safety?* Are electrical outlets covered? Is there a fire extinguisher and a smoke detector?
- *What provisions are made for snacks and lunches for the children?* Do they have menus that you can review? Can you sample the food yourself?
- *Policies.* What do they do if a child becomes ill? What about very ill—needing emergency treatment right away?
- *How do they discipline children?* Do they have a policy on corporal punishment (hitting or spanking)? If they allow corporal punishment, avoid them. Sometimes angry people hit harder than they intend to.
- *Staff credentials.* Does the facility run criminal records checks on all staff members? (Do not automatically assume that they do.)
- *Is the facility licensed?* Look at the license to see how current it is. It should be posted in a prominent place.
- *Facility credentials.* Is it accredited by any national or state organizations?

The National Resource Center for Health and Safety in Childcare recommends these staff-to-child ratios in childcare centers:

Age of Child	Child-to-Staff Ratio	Maximum No. of Children in Group
0 to 12 months	3 to 1	6
13 to 24 months	3 to 1	6
25 to 30 months	4 to 1	8
35 to 36 months	5 to 1	10
3 years	7 to 1	14
4 years	8 to 1	16
5 years	8 to 1	16
6 to 8 years	10 to 1	20
9 to 12 years	12 to 1	24

Bad Facilities

You also need to know what kind of features constitutes a bad childcare center. Here are some key factors that should alert you to inherent problems:

- There's no warmth between the caregivers and children.
- There are obvious health or safety violations, such as no safety latches on windows, no disinfectant spray by the changing table, or cleaning products within easy reach of children.

- Parents are made to feel unwelcome. When you drop off your child or pick her up, you feel like an intruder or an annoyance.
- The caregiver-child ratio has been exceeded, and it's clear there is no plan to hire more workers.

ON TIME TO PICK UP YOUR CHILD?

Be sure to find out each childcare facility's policy about lateness, if you have a tendency to be late. Ann Douglas says that some facilities charge as much as $1.00 for every *minute* you're late. If you're supposed to pick up your child at 5 P.M. and you arrive at 5:15, then you'll owe $15. That can add up!

Although you can't expect childcare centers to watch your child until you feel like arriving, take a hard look at the policies and penalties for lateness. If you're in the kind of job that regularly forces you to be late, find out if the lateness policy could be negotiable. Rather than paying the late fee every time, could you find a creative arrangement for you bartering or giving the center something it needs? Food, storybooks, something else? Brainstorm ideas!

No matter how effective you are at negotiation, if you are constantly late, sometimes you'll be forced to pay extra fees. If your main problem is losing track of time, get an alarm watch that you can set ten minutes (or some other timeframe that works for you) before you must leave work to pick up your child.

▶ IS YOUR JOB ADD-UNFRIENDLY?

Another consideration, affecting both your children as well as yourself, is whether your job is what I call "ADD-friendly." I don't mean a job that allows you to do whatever you want and whenever you feel like it. But I am referring to a job that encourages creativity over rigid structure and that appreciates the intelligence and ability of most women with ADD.

What kind of job is that? An artist or writer? Or maybe an advertising executive or police officer? It need not be "artsy" to make a mom with ADD happy. Other factors come into play: For example, a secretary may think her job is ADD-friendly because her boss is understanding about her need for frequent breaks and switching from task to task. Or the general environment may feel positive: It could be an office where an employee feels if she is a little late or if she misplaces some papers and needs to search for them, no one will become terribly upset.

If you are very unhappy in your job and feel it is not a match for your personality, and your ADD is constantly causing you to fall backward, it may be a good idea to think about changing careers.

When the Job Environment Is Good

When your job is a good fit for you as a person with ADD, then half the battle is won. Many women with ADD find success with jobs that don't constrict them and that allow them to celebrate their individuality and their creativity. You may need some accommodations, such as reminders to stay on task, or written rather than verbal instructions, or both. But if you're receiving these accommodations and they enable you to be effective at your job, then you're in an ADD-friendly job environment.

So how does your job environment fit? Consider these responses from Moms with ADD:

- I'm a customer service employee and it's friendly. My job is varied, not repetitive, and it's also interesting. I'm good at working with people, terrible at paperwork.
- I am a manager of a doctor's office. It's friendly. I have the freedom to walk around whenever I want, and there are varieties of things to do that don't take a lot of time. Parts of this job require more discipline to get done what needs to get done, and I find it hard to do these until the last minute when the adrenaline rush kicks in. My director is aware of my ADD, as is everyone in the office.
- I am a shipping specialist and it's so-so. I mostly work independently and this helps. More praise and positive feedback would be better.
- I'm an artist—definitely ADD-friendly. I make my own hours—the hard part is recordkeeping.
- My job is in the marketing and administrative field: so-so. The marketing is friendly, but the administrative/accounting side is not.

When There Are Problems

Sometimes the job environment is *not* good. You may be in a job that is too rigid for you. Your creativity may be seen as an annoying problem rather than a great asset, because you're expected to behave in certain specific ways at certain specific times; and no deviations are accepted. Perhaps being on time is extremely important and you have a lot of trouble with punctuality.

You may need to think seriously about changing jobs or even your career. It is possible to change, even if you think you are "too old." I knew a woman who received her social-work degree at age 70. What did she do then? She got a job as a social worker. She also started thinking about getting a master's in social work.

Don't tell me it will take you three or more years to get your degree, because I will then say to you, "How old will you be in three years if you don't get your degree?"

Sometimes the workplace can be modified to accommodate some of your ADD symptoms, and that accommodation alone will be sufficient to enable you to perform your job well. Read the last section of this chapter, which discusses laws about the workplace. And also know that you don't necessarily have to invoke a particular law to your employer in order to request a change. Many workers simply tell their boss, "I have a problem with this noise level and it's hard for me to concentrate. Is it okay if I work with earphones on to drown out the noise?" Most employers won't have a problem with such a request.

▶ WORK IS STILL THERE WHEN YOU'RE AT HOME

Some moms report that when they are at work, they can *only* think of work and their family may as well not exist. They focus all their brain's energy on work. Conversely, when they are at home, the workplace ceases to exist. Yet often there are some things that you need to do about home while at work (like make your child a doctor's appointment) and some work things you need to do while at home—such as call a coworker who didn't come in today to remind him that the big meeting is tomorrow.

Other moms report that they worry about their children while at work, and they worry about their job when they're at home. They can never fully be in one place or the other. If a woman feels more comfortable that she has a system set in place to cover both bases, then she's also less likely to worry about the place where she's not.

A solution to help mothers with both kinds of problems could be to write yourself notes or set up reminders. Another possibility is to set aside time at lunch to handle doctor or dentist appointment calls and other home matters. Do be sure, however, that once in awhile you enjoy lunch with a friend. This is important for your emotional health!

Writing Yourself Notes

If you can't call about your child's dentist appointment when you're at home—because the dentist's office is closed by then—you'll need to make the call at work. A note to yourself in your dayplanner, calendar, or whatever items you take back and forth from work to home can solve that problem.

Write yourself notes to resolve work issues that must be handled when you are at home, in a similar manner. Although you should try to keep your two "worlds" separate, sometimes worlds collide in the "wrong" timeframe. So if you will need to make a call or finish a report at home, write it down.

Setting Up Reminders

Don't expect yourself to keep track in your head of all the many goings-on of you and your family members. It's too hard! Instead, set up reminders for yourself, whether it's something you hear (calling yourself up on your own phone answering machine), it's visual (something you are forced to see, such as notes to yourself), or you set up reminders on your computer. You can also use several types of reminder systems so you have emergency backup reminders.

1. You may also wish to list important tasks on your Palm Pilot or other portable or laptop computer. Many say they could not function without these devices to help them keep track of their responsibilities and alert them to upcoming appointments, deadlines, and other important events.

2. Call your home or office and leave yourself a message to be sure to do such-and-such. Sounds silly, but it works!

3. To keep your family in mind while at work, consider family photographs or drawings that your children make. Often the sight of your child's face or her drawing may trigger the memory that you are supposed to do something related to your family.

I'm not suggesting you keep a photo of your boss at home. But you might hang up or tape up something that reminds you of work when you're at home—such as an award you received or a friendly card from your fellow workers. Seeing these items can help trigger you to remember to take a work action while at home.

▶ LAWS THAT AFFECT WORKERS TODAY

Citing the Americans with Disabilities Act, a Nevada couple complained that a childcare center would no longer provide childcare to their daughter because of her attention deficit disorder, according to a 1999 U.S. Department of Justice report, "Enforcing the ADA." The owner of the center agreed to comply with the ADA and provide services to the child and train her staff.

Several key laws are important for women to know about. If you're a mom with ADD, you may find one or more of these laws helpful to you in struggles you face in the workplace. In this section, I'll briefly discuss two major laws that could affect you: the Family and Medical Leave Act and the Americans with Disabilities Act.

The Family and Medical Leave Act

The Family and Medical Leave Act, passed in 1993, allows for up to twelve weeks of unpaid time off for your illness or the illness of a family member.

If your children, spouse, or elderly parents become ill and need care, you can provide that care and not fear that you'll get fired. You will need to notify your employer and follow the provisions of the law. The law also covers adoptive parents.

The Americans with Disabilities Act

The Americans with Disabilities Act of 1990 requires employers to accommodate workers with disabilities. Whether your ADD is a "disability" depends upon how severe your particular ADD is, the type of job you are in, and the accommodations you think that you need, to name a few considerations. If you think that you are being discriminated against, you may wish to consult an attorney to find out if your case is worth pursuing.

Some accommodations can be made on your own. For others, you may need a supervisor's permission to make changes. Some workers bring in white-noise machines to block out distractions, and unless it drives your office mate completely crazy, this is an accommodation you should be able to make on your own.

An example of an accommodation that you might request is a change in the lighting. Fluorescent lights that periodically blink and flicker may drive you wild. If so, request a change to long-persistence phosphor lighting. These tubes will greatly reduce the flickering problem. They may cost slightly more but generally last longer.

The U.S. Department of Justice offers a toll-free line with information about the Americans with Disabilities Act. Specialists answer questions from 10 A.M. Eastern Time to 6 P.M. on Mondays, Tuesdays, Wednesdays, and Fridays. On Thursday, the line is available from 1 P.M. to 6 P.M. Call 800-514-0301.

Juggling the demands of both your family and your job can be extremely challenging for anyone, and even more so for the mother with ADD. In this chapter, I covered issues such as finding good childcare so you can feel secure while at work, considering whether your job is ADD-friendly, and understanding basic laws that protect you.

PART TWO

Family Matters

The challenges of parenting vary depending on whether your child is an infant, schoolage child or teenager. For the mom with ADD there are unique challenges at each stage. It's also true that the family dynamic is affected if your children also have ADD. Sometimes non-ADD children feel shortchanged. This part covers the many issues involved in parenting for the mom with ADD.

6

Your Children Have ADD—Or Don't

All families are different, including families with moms who have ADD. Some families include children who also have ADD, and some are comprised of children who don't have ADD. Or there may be some children with ADD and other non-ADD kids. A further complicating factor can be the significant other or husband. Whether Dad has ADD also greatly influences the entire family dynamic.

In this chapter, you'll learn ways of handling life with ADD in the following situations:

- When your children have ADD too
- When your children don't have ADD
- When some of your children have ADD and some don't

▶ YOUR CHILDREN HAVE ADD TOO

If you're a mom with ADD, the odds are pretty high—as much as 70 percent—that your child will have ADD too. The genetic link is pretty clearly established. Since you have no control over your genes, it's not your fault if your child inherited a predisposition toward ADD. However, some adoptive moms have ADD—as do children they adopted.

Sometimes It's Harder when the Kids Have ADD Too

Although she did not study whether the mothers had ADD, in one interesting study Merle Langbord Levine, M.Ed., of the Merle Levine Academy, Inc., in Toronto, Ontario, looked at mothers with more than one child and at least one child with ADD. She compared the mother's parenting in various aspects to the ADD child and the non-ADD child. The sample was small but the findings are intriguing.

Levine studied 15 upper-middle-class women, most of whom (67 percent) were college graduates. She found that in parenting a child with ADD there was a significant impact on the mother herself in the form of greater emotional stress, more physical illnesses, and more instances of anger—versus the impact on the mother of parenting a non-ADD child. Levine also said, "The study suggests that mothers of ADHD children bear the brunt of the blame for their ADHD child's problems and behaviour."

The study revealed that prior to the diagnosis of the child, expenses were much higher for the child with ADD (50 percent greater); and the mothers were harsher as well as less consistent in disciplining the child with ADD, often because of the mother's exhaustion. In some cases, mothers were so stressed out that they canceled planned outings with the child. Feelings of guilt and helplessness were high; the marital relationship was also negatively affected because of intense disagreements and arguments between husbands and wives.

A pretty grim picture—but there is some good news here! Levine also looked at how the mother fared *before* the child was diagnosed versus *after* diagnosis, and the situation was greatly changed. Said Levine,

> A major finding, following the child's diagnosis and implementation of medication, is that the mother's guilt is relieved and she is able to reframe the disorder in more rational, positive ways. The issue of blame (on the mother) is virtually extinguished, and the mother is then free to deal more constructively with her ADHD child and her/his myriad of problems. The diagnosis is found to be crucial for the mother's well-being and is also the impetus for empowering her to seek out the most effective behavioural and academic rehabilitation services for her child. As well, all of the mothers reported a positive improvement in their marital relationships and report that their husbands became more supportive of them. At the same time the mothers indicated that their relationship with extended family members also improved.

Levine also found that, desite the diagnosis, the mothers did need to continue actively advocating for their children in the schools.

Many of the women I interviewed said they suspected that one child had ADD, but they weren't sure. They thought they would wait until the child was schoolage and not take any action until then. Based on Levine's study, it seems that it would be far more prudent for mothers diagnosed with ADD themselves to seek diagnosis of their children who they believe may have ADD. It would seem a good course of action not only for the mother, but for the child.

Helping Your Child Get Diagnosed and Treated

Many parents actually discover their own ADD after their child has been diagnosed. When they hear about the basic symptoms—the inattentiveness, impulsivity, and so forth, often parents have an "Aha" moment when it occurs to them that this may actually explain all the trouble they've had for so many years.

But in fewer cases, the parent is diagnosed with ADD first and the children may come second. Or perhaps neither of you have been diagnosed, and you strongly *suspect* that you and your children have ADD. If you do, it's a very good idea to get your child professional help before or during elementary school. Many kids with ADD can manage to pull themselves through grades kindergarten through six, but when it comes to middle school or junior high and then high school, the academic and social demands become far greater. It's good if you have a support system in place before then.

But if your child isn't diagnosed until he's a teenager, do not despair. There are still many things that therapists, the school, and you can do to help your adolescent during these often-difficult years.

Getting Your Child to Take Medication

If your child is diagnosed with ADD, you can expect that most physicians will wish to try an ADD-specific medication like Ritalin or Dexedrine or another medicine. Several problems often occur when a parent is given a prescription for medication to treat her ADD child. Here are some common reactions, no matter how reassuring the doctor is:

- The mother is fearful of using medication and delays or doesn't fill a prescription.
- The mother fills the prescription but gives the medicine to her child with great trepidation. She anxiously watches for any awful symptoms or side effects.
- The mother worries that she is a bad mother who is "drugging out" her child, or she hears from others that it's bad to give a child "drugs."

ARE YOU *OVER*-IDENTIFYING WITH YOUR CHILD WHO HAS ADD?

It's important to recognize the boundaries between you and your child in order to give him or her what is needed. This can be difficult sometimes, when you see your child struggle with ADD symptoms that you faced yourself as a child. Here's why:

- You may think you know exactly how your child feels. Maybe you're right. But you could be completely wrong. And what might have helped you could be the wrong answer for your child.

- You may over-identify with your child and as a result, try to make things too easy for him or her. Sure, it's hard to see a child have similar problems. But you couldn't learn to walk for your child, and there will be some emotional tripping—and getting up and moving on. Don't thwart that process.

- If you over-identify, you could become trapped in a fearful mindset—"My childhood was miserable, and I'm going to make it different for my child." This is good if you direct this energy toward advocating for your child. But it's bad if you convey your own fears to the child.

Symptoms of Over-Identification

- You are spending hours on your child's homework every night, and you're exhausted.
- You see "yourself" or ADD in every problem your child has.
- You give in to your child's requests out of guilt.
- You make extraordinary allowances for your child, because he has ADD.

If You're Afraid to Give Your Child Meds

It's easy to be scared by media claims that too many people are drugging their children and to feel that there must be a better way: a different diet, different parenting techniques, a new therapist—*something*. However, clinical research on children and adults with ADD indicates that medication is an important adjunct to treatment.

Therapy alone can accomplish little, because it's too hard for your child to pay attention or to remember what advice the therapist offered, no matter how good the therapist. Therapy can be helpful, however, when used in conjunction with medication. There is no medical evidence or other evidence than anecdotal reports that changing a child's diet will do any good at all.

Sugar does not cause ADD. If you remove or cut back sugar from a child's diet, the ADD won't go away. You may think you see an improvement, and a large part of this is that often we see what we want to see. But over the long term, improvements are rarely found by changes in a child's diet.

What about supplemental vitamins, herbs, or other "natural" treatments? Because of insufficient clinical trials, the jury is still out on whether they work. It is possible they may help. But remember these are still drugs, even if they are natural, and even if they are non-prescription. Cobra venom is also natural. There is a huge range of products and items that are natural, and some are helpful and others are not.

It's not bad to be a careful and cautious mother, no matter what medication you are administering. It's a good idea to learn ahead of time what possible side effects could occur, and what you should be watching out for.

Don't assume that the medication will hurt your child. It may not do much of anything at all, or it may help your child. You should also be sure to ask the doctor if it is a fast-acting medication, so you would see changes quickly or a more slow-acting medication that requires days or weeks before its cumulative effect really "kicks in" and provides its full efficacy to the child.

If You Think You're Bad to Give Your Child Drugs

It's not surprising that many parents worry about giving their children drugs, especially the stimulants that are usually prescribed to treat ADD. Newspaper and magazine articles and hysterical newscasters on TV warn darkly of parents who are drugging their children, robbing them of their childhood. It can appear that the parent who allows or encourages her child to take medication is not doing her best as a parent, or is even being a bad parent.

There are also specific religious and other groups who have a particular aversion to psychiatric medications. It appears their new favorite drug to hate is Ritalin, and it's easy to stimulate fear and blame because it's a medication given to children.

But let me ask you this: If your child has an ear infection, are you evil if you give him the antibiotic your pediatrician prescribes? If your daughter has epilepsy, is it wrong to give her anti-epilepsy medication so she can avoid having seizures?

If your answer is that it's okay to give children medications in these circumstances, then why is it wrong to give a child with ADD a medication that can help that child concentrate and focus better, and help that child improve her school performance? In my mind, a good parent considers the various possibilities; and if an ADD medication appears to be indicated, then she will have her child try that medication. In doing so, she will be carefully observing her child for any possible side effects and other problem areas for people with ADD, as well as looking for improvements in her child's concentration.

Lies, Damn Lies, and Statistics

It is easy to misunderstand or purposely misuse statistics, and that is often what happens when the conversation turns to the number or percentage of children taking Ritalin.

Let me give you an example. What if I told you that use of Ritalin by high school children more than *tripled* from 1975 to 1993? Oh, no! But you might feel differently if you learned more facts: The percentage of high school students taking Ritalin in 1975 was .22 percent (less than 1 percent), and that rate increased to .70 in 1993 (still less than 1 percent).

This statistic, and many others like it, was reported in the February 1, 2000, issue of the *Journal of the American Academy of Child and Adolescent Psychiatry,* which reviewed studies on children taking Ritalin. The researchers found that studies have revealed many children with ADD are undermedicated. In some areas, only 25 percent of children meeting the diagnostic criteria for attention deficit disorder were taking medication.

They also found disparities in *who* was receiving medication; for example, African American children were about half as likely to receive Ritalin than White children. Boys were more likely to receive it than girls. The authors concluded,

> Stimulant treatments are prescribed with greater frequency than 10 years ago and are obtained by about two thirds of children with ADHD at some point in their childhood; however, the availability and use of stimulants varies substantially by geographic region and also seems to be influenced by gender and race.

Perhaps there should be an outcry: Not *enough* children are getting the help they need.

Helping Your Child with Organization

Most moms with ADD have a very difficult time with organization. So it's like "the blind leading the blind" when it comes to helping your child with organization.

ORGANIZE BY DONATING OLD TOYS TO CHARITY

Does your child have plenty of old toys that he or she clings to, but are just adding to the clutter in the bedroom? Claudia Taskier, a professional organizer in Washington, D.C., says that rather than fighting, why not ask your child if he or she would like to donate old toys to a child who doesn't have them? It's a lot nicer and easier for a child to think of giving a doll or fire truck to a child who has no toys than it is to think of it in the trash can. Such a strategy also empowers your child.

But a key advantage of having ADD yourself is that you understand what it feels like from the inside, and you may exhibit many of the same symptoms that your child shows. You have a head start with the empathy factor, and that's very helpful.

Next, as you learn methods of organizing and strategies to help you remember to do things, you can also teach your child what you've learned. You may not want to rush out and buy him a vibrating watch. But you may find that an alarm clock would be helpful, and you may find other options as well. Thus, you can adapt what you've learned to help your child handle his or her ADD better.

One good idea, in addition to reading books by experts, is to ask your child's therapist for advice on dealing with disciplinary problems with your child. It's also a very good idea to tell the therapist that you have ADD yourself, so that you can devise strategies that are workable for you and will be effective for your child.

When Your Child Has Other Problems on Top of ADD

Experts say that as many as one-third or more of the children with ADD have a "co-morbid" disorder. This means that in addition to the ADD, another problem occurs at the same time. It could be a problem such as depression, anxiety, or another mood disorder, like bipolar disorder (manic depression). It could also be a behavioral problem, such as oppositional-defiant disorder or even conduct disorder.

Many people think that children cannot suffer from severely debilitating mood disorders such as clinical depression, anxiety, or bipolar disorder. After all, they're children, they are supposed to be carefree and let the adults solve all the world's problems. It would be nice if children didn't suffer from depression, but the fact is that sometimes they do. Some children are so ill with clinical depression that they actually commit suicide or cause serious harm to themselves. No child who threatens suicide should be scoffed at, no matter how young they are.

If a child with ADD also suffers from depression, the good news is that depression is highly treatable with medication and with therapy. Some antidepressants, such as Wellbutrin (buproprion) are also used to treat ADD. In addition, when a child is being treated with a stimulant medication such as Ritalin, it can often be supplemented with an antidepressant medication, and there are many different types of antidepressants. Therapy may also be helpful to the child and to the family.

There are also medications that can help with the rages of bipolar disorder. Experts say bipolar disorder does not present as euphoria and depression in children, as it does in adults. Instead, the "manic" portion of bipolar disorder can be seen in severe rages children exhibit, in which they destroy things on purpose versus the accidental destruction that can ensue from ADD. Some experts believe some children diagnosed with ADD actually have an early case of bipolar disorder. This is important because the medication for bipolar disorder may be different from what is prescribed for ADD.

Siblings of Children with ADD

Studies of the biological siblings of children with ADD have revealed that there is an increased probability of seeing ADD in the siblings of children diagnosed with ADD. In a study published in 2000 in *Genetic Epidemiology*, researchers Stephen Faraone, Joseph Biederman, and Michael Monuteaux studied 140 children diagnosed with attention deficit hyperactivity disorder and 120 non-ADHD children.

They found that when the child had ADHD, the risk was 20 percent that siblings would also have ADHD. The risk for non-ADHD children having siblings with ADHD was 5 percent. They also looked at some co-morbidities and found, for example, that if a child were diagnosed with ADHD and bipolar disorder (BPD), there was a nearly 56 percent risk that siblings would also have these disorders. The risk for the non-ADHD/non-BPD siblings was 5 percent.

The study also looked at the risk of parents having ADHD when their children were diagnosed with the disorder. They found the rate was nearly 15 percent for the parents of children with ADHD and about 3 percent for the parents of the non-ADHD children. When the child was diagnosed with both ADHD and bipolar disorder, the risk was about 36 percent that the parents also presented with these two diagnoses.

These statistics are probably not an artifact of the environment; that is, living with a person with ADD does not induce the same condition in the rest of the household. Adoption studies have shown that the rate of ADD in adopted children is related to the rate in their birth, not their adoptive families.

Of course, it's important to take a hard look at the other side of these statistics. For example, although there's a 20 percent risk that the siblings of children with ADHD will also have ADHD, there are also 80 percent of siblings who do *not* have ADHD. And of that 15 percent of parents who have ADHD when their children are diagnosed with ADHD, there are also 85% who do not have ADHD. As a result, most of the siblings and parents of children with ADHD do not have attention deficit disorder, based on current studies.

▶ **YOUR CHILDREN DON'T HAVE ADD**

"My daughter doesn't have ADD and sometimes she gets so frustrated with me. But long ago, she figured out how to compensate!" says Ellen, 41, mother of a daughter who is now ten years old. "When she was little, about six years old, she'd get into bed and ask me to read her a story. I'd tell her I'd be there in fifteen minutes . . . well, that time came and went and she fell asleep."

Continues Ellen, "This smart little girl created her own strategy. She would come to me in the kitchen and say, Mommy, come read me a story. I'd stay 'I will in fifteen minutes.' Then she said, 'Okay, Mommy, I'm setting the kitchen timer for fifteen minutes so you don't forget.' And you know what? It worked!"

ARE YOU *UNDER*-IDENTIFYING WITH YOUR NON-ADD CHILD?

Some moms with ADD under-identify with their children who do *not* have ADD, and this can be problematic as well. Rather than over-identifying with the child, they may feel detached. Here are some possible indicators of under-identifying with a child:

- The child pleads for help, but you don't think the problem is that big a deal. He should handle it himself. You may be right. Each situation should be considered. The problem lies in ignoring *all* requests for help. This is a common mistake. Many moms with ADD think their children can handle anything.

- Your child's grades are falling, but you assume everything will be okay since he's basically an organized kind of person.

Challenges of Parenting the Non-ADD Child

Although the non-ADD child is usually calmer and often does not require as much attention as the child with ADD, it isn't necessarily easier to raise a non-ADD child. One reason is that the mother and child may become frustrated with the great differences in how they look at the world and how they operate in it.

In addition, as illustrated earlier, it isn't so easy to be the *child* of the mom with ADD. "They often end up not trusting your memory or judgment and sometimes use your self-doubt to their advantage," said Maria, 32, mother of three school-age children.

Other mothers agree that parenting the non-ADD child is more challenging than people realize. "I know I see things differently and my order of how things should be done may seem backwards to others. My daughter finds it hard to understand the way I do things and often gets very frustrated with me," says Rhonda, 36, mother of a teenager.

Non-ADD Children Who "Parentalize"

Sometimes children of moms with ADD try to take on grown-up roles because they don't think that Mom is handling the details adequately, or at all. The potential danger is that although such behavior may seem positive or cute to Mom and to others, it can also be a negative for a child to take on adult roles.

Why? Because children don't have the experience or judgment to make adult decisions, and they should not be put in that position. Even though it can be tough for the mother with ADD, it's up to Mom to make the major decisions. Sometimes the parentalizing isn't severe, but it's still uncomfortable for the mother. For example, if your non-ADD child is constantly reminding you to be *sure* to pick him up, or complaining about your not doing the laundry yet again, the common response is anger and annoyance.

Says psychologist and ADD expert Kathleen Nadeau, "The appropriate response is for Mom to acknowledge, you're right, I did forget to pick you up last time. I promise I will remember to pick you up and here's what I will do to make sure that I remember." She can then show the child her calendar where she has written it down.

Another example: the dirty laundry. Nadeau says Mom could say, "You're right, I didn't get the laundry done. I had a really tough week but why don't we work on it together?" In these examples, the mother is accepting her responsibility, but she is also acting like an adult too.

Following are some examples of children who are exhibiting parentalizing behavior that is troubling.

1. **The child self-administers medication.** I am not talking about your teenager getting herself an aspirin, after telling you that she has a headache and plans to do this. I am talking about parents who expect their children not only to get their own medicine, but even to dispense medication to other children or adults in the family. This is a very bad idea, whether we are talking about aspirin or Ritalin.

Children don't have the experience or judgment to dispense medication. They probably won't read the bottle. The pharmacy directions printed on the bottle may be to take half a pill, but they'll take a whole pill. Children also tend to think "more is better." Thus, they may reason, I feel really bad, so I should take five aspirins. This kind of thinking can be dangerous or even lethal.

It's also psychologically bad for minor children to dispense medication, because this is a power that should be reserved for adults only. In addition, because of youth and a tendency to magical thinking, a child may come to think of taking medication as an easy way to get better fast, or the solution to all problems. He may also assume that he is more powerful or knowledgeable than he really is.

2. **The child gets mom medication.** When a minor is expected to get Mom her medication, this act is putting the child in a pseudo-parental role and Mom in a pseudo-child role. It can diminish the child's view of Mom's authority and competency. Mom is the sick person and I am the competent person who is helping take care of Sick Mom. I am stronger than Mom is.

3. **The child does most or all of the cooking and cleaning.** Children should not be doing most of the cooking and cleaning, because children—although they

should have jobs around the house—should also be engaged in homework and in playtime. If they are spending all their free time keeping the house in shape, they are being robbed of their childhood, and their grades could also suffer as a result.

4. **The child makes all or most of the decisions about how the weekend will be spent.** Certainly your children's wishes about what to do on the weekend, vacations, and so forth should be heard. But when a child calls all the shots about what the family will do this weekend, and the parents go meekly along with the child's wishes, this child has far too much power and the parents are far too passive.

Your Non-ADD Children Need You

Some moms see their non-ADD children as so effectual that they forget that everybody—including non-ADD children—has problems sometimes and needs advice and/or sympathy. But even if Larry always gets his homework done on time and has a room so clean an Army drill sergeant would be impressed, he still sometimes is worried about problems and needs your help. Even smart, competent children need their mothers.

Here are some points to keep in mind when parenting your non-ADD children:

- Make special alone time for you and the child, at least once a week. A walk, a movie, roller skating. The togetherness is more important than the activity.
- Find common ground. Instead of constantly thinking about how different you are, consider ways you are alike or similar. This can help draw you together.
- Don't always take the side of your child with ADD, and don't expect these children to work it out all the time. Intervention may be needed.
- Help your non-ADD child connect with other adults who don't have ADD, such as friends or relatives.

Classic Problems with the Non-ADD Child

Here are some examples of classic problems that you may already have seen in your non-ADD child. You should note that similar behaviors may be found when one child in the family receives an extraordinary amount of attention because of a physical or emotional problem or developmental delay.

1. **Mimics ADD-like behavior to get attention.** Parents should not be shocked if their non-ADD child exhibits ADD-like behavior. If that's what works to get attention, the child may scream, refuse to obey, and mimic other behaviors of the child with ADD.

2. **Maintains a low (too low) profile.** Because of the high drama that the child with ADD may also present with, the non-ADD child may react by staying away from the other child or even from the family itself. Lonely and reclusive, he may repress his problems and not seek out help he needs.

3. **Tries to be perfect.** Because the non-ADD child can do many things that the ADD child has trouble with, parents tend to assume that she is competent at everything—or could be, if she only tried hard enough. Thus, we can fall into the classic trap that aggravates us so much when other people assume that *we* could do just fine if we worked hard. The child herself may buy into this myth.

No matter how smart or "good" your non-ADD child is, it's impossible for her to excel at everything. Once in awhile, the child will find herself faltering and needing parental help and guidance, or at least some sympathy for the problems that she faces.

4. **Doesn't tell you about problems.** Don't think non-ADD children never have problems: they do. Just because they do well in school, can remember not only to do their homework but actually bring it back to school too (unlike your child with ADD), this does not mean life is always easy.

▶ SOME OF YOUR CHILDREN HAVE ADD—AND SOME DON'T

"It's not that I neglected my child who didn't have ADD. He got baths, food, etc. But I had to spend so much time with my daughter who had ADD until she went on Ritalin. I mean I would spend eight hours a day doing nothing but cleaning up a terrorist attack on the Lego bricks, then have to move on to whatever crashed in the other room. I'd also often have to bandage a constantly moving child," said Sandy, 39, mother of a teenage son and daughter.

"But my son could entertain himself. He is a quiet child. All he wanted once in awhile was for me to read him a story after she finally went to sleep, and I would literally fall asleep while reading him the story. At three years of age, he would cover me with a blanket, turn out the light, and go to sleep himself. Talk about Guilt with a capital G!"

Parents who themselves have ADD may sometimes over-identify with their child who has ADD too. "Although I get frustrated with my child with ADD, I find I understand what makes him 'tick' much better. It's often hard for me to understand the 'why' behind my younger non-ADD son's behavior," says Trish, 32, mother of two sons.

Key Issues with Non-ADD Siblings

Although very few studies have been done on families who have children with and without ADD, one important study was reported on in a 1999 issue of *Family Process* by professor and researcher Judy Kendall.

Some problems that Kendall identified in the non-ADD siblings she studied were

- Being expected to be good and nearly "invisible"
- Given too much responsibility for their ADD sibling

- Parents not believing non-ADD children who reported on physical aggression that their ADD siblings used on them
- Feelings that life was chaotic and would never get better

The Invisible Non-ADD Child

Because of the chaos a child with ADD can cause, to both non-ADD moms and mothers with ADD, often a great deal of time and effort is expended on the child with ADD. As illustrated in the beginning of this chapter, the mother with ADD may be so exhausted from her efforts with her child who has ADD that she has little time or energy left for her other children. She may not even notice if and when they are experiencing problems.

In addition, non-ADD children have reported that even when they have difficult problems or worries, their parents may minimize them and tell them not to worry about it, thus not validating the child's own concerns. Several probable causes for Mom's behavior may be that the ADD behavior seems so difficult that "normal" problems seem trivial in comparison. Another possibility is that the non-ADD child is seen as so competent that he "should" be able to handle problems. And yet children who don't have ADD can face difficulties in school and at home and have trouble sorting out how to deal with them.

Non-ADD Siblings Given Too Much Responsibility

Another common problem is that overburdened mothers may give the non-ADD child responsibility for many tasks that are typically handled by parents. In the study reported in the professional journal *Family Process,* non-ADD children were expected to take care of lunch money for their younger and older siblings, watch out for them in general, and even to handle such parental tasks as administering medication.

When non-ADD siblings are given too much responsibility for their siblings with ADD, they may become resentful, angry, or even clinically depressed. Kendall also found that although parents expected much of non-ADD siblings in the caregiving of their siblings who have ADD, at the same time the non-ADD children were given very little power and were rarely asked for their input. Thus, they had accountability and responsibility—but no input. This would be very frustrating for a person of any age.

Parents Not Listening to Reports of Aggression

He hits me every day. He just all of a sudden hauls off and hits me all of a sudden. I don't know why. My Mom says it's a part of his hyperactivity. My Mom tells me not to worry about it, that it will get better. I don't see how. The other day he sat on me and it was hard to breathe. But I know that if I fight him back it will be worse. So I try to wait it out. I worry sometimes that he might kill me. I know he wouldn't mean to, but I think it could happen.

8-year-old, non-ADD child, speaking about his 13-year-old
brother with ADD (*Family Process,* Spring 1999)

One very serious problem that sometimes occurs between siblings when some have ADD and others do not is the risk for aggressive behavior; and sometimes that behavior can be severe. Kendall's study indicated that parents tended to minimize or even disbelieve a child when he or she reported being attacked by a sibling with ADD. This is a distressing finding: No child should be physically abused by other children in the family, despite their disabilities.

If your non-ADD child complains of being attacked, don't make these mistakes:

1. Assuming the non-ADD child is lying or exaggerating. He probably is not. Even if he is stretching the truth, you should investigate first before making this assumption.

2. Assuming that fighting is "normal" for a child with ADD and there's just nothing you can do about. Some children with ADD have reported that they could get away with far more serious abuse when it was perpetrated on a sibling than they could ever get away with if they did the same thing to someone in school.

3. Assuming that a parent is helpless to stop the abuse. You are not helpless and you must intervene. It could become necessary to involve law enforcement personnel if the attacks are serious. In one case that I know about, the anger of one teenage girl became so intense that one night she actually stabbed her older brother in the chest with a butcher knife. She meant to kill. Fortunately, her aim was bad and he was injured but recovered. At that point, law enforcement involvement was mandatory.

Remember, if you are tacitly abetting abuse by your inaction, there is also the possibility that you could be charged with "neglect" for allowing reported abuse to continue. In some cases, the state protective services removed children from the family because of such neglect and placed them in foster homes.

4. Assuming that physical aggression is a "normal" part of sibling rivalry. Although it is true that siblings jockey for positions of favor with their parents, physical abuse—particularly on a regular basis—is not normal. It must be stopped. If you feel or find that you cannot control the abusive behavior and actions of one child taken against another child, then it's imperative that you seek professional advice from a psychiatrist, psychologist, or other person. You need to act in the best interests of all your children, and you are doing the abusive child no favors by allowing the abuse to continue. It is not unreasonable to allow the non-ADD child to have a lock on his door, if that will make him feel safe.

Feeling Life Is Chaotic and Will Never Improve

Some non-ADD children report that they never know what the child with ADD will do next, and they can never really look forward to any event. They feel resigned and even depressed. It's very important for parents to actually "see" their non-ADD children. Instead of concentrating on guilt for having ignored the child in the past, take time to talk to the non-ADD child regularly—and without the child with ADD tagging along.

Your child with ADD may greatly resent this and do everything he or she can to disrupt plans to be with the non-ADD sibling(s), but it's important to create a plan to help your non-ADD children have special time with you too.

Whether or not your child has ADD too can make a big difference in how you parent a child. The mother with ADD may over-identify with the child who has ADD, and she may under-identify with the non-ADD child. She may also have unreasonably high expectations of the non-ADD child, assuming he has no problems since he doesn't have ADD. It's also true that sometimes when some children have ADD and others do not, this interaction can be a problem. I addressed these issues and others in this chapter.

7

You Have a Baby: But What If You Have ADD Too?

It's very exciting to have your first child, or even your fourth child! Babies are wonderful creatures. They are also dependent individuals who rely on their mothers or other caregivers for their very survival. They need you for food, shelter, clothing, love, protection, and limits. Most of these are self-evident: nutritious food and enough of it; clothing that is warm or cool enough and comfortable; a home where they feel safe.

This chapter provides practical advice for the mom with ADD who is parenting an infant or toddler, including:

- Basics about babies and toddler
- Limits with love
- Your own expectations of yourself as a new mother

▶ BABIES/TODDLERS

Most new mothers find that the 24-hour nature of being a new mother is very daunting. It doesn't end at 5 or 6 P.M., or when you go to bed at night. You're always Mom and you're always "on." There's a multitude of decisions to make and sometimes not much time to make them. Sometimes ADD is a distinct advantage, because if you are impulsive and you see your baby or child in danger, you may react faster than the non-ADD mom, who needs time to process what's going on. You don't. You act.

Jenny, now age 32, relates the problems she faced and the major lessons that she has learned from them.

"My ADD is of the non-hyperactive variety. For me, that means that I need a lot of down time. I also crave quiet and calm. If you have been blessed with a sweet-tempered, easy baby, you are indeed lucky. My babies were not 'easy' babies. One had colic for three months. The other didn't sleep through the night till she was seven months old. Which brings me to what I consider one of the toughest parts for an ADD mom when it comes to babies: lack of sleep!

"Without enough sleep, everything bothers me a lot. Couple that with having to attend to a baby's needs twenty-four hours a day, and you can have yourself one monster of a mother. When my firstborn needed to be carried around constantly because of colic, I really despaired. She had such a piercing cry, it was painful to hear. My hypersensitivity, which I wasn't aware of then, made living with a screaming baby even more challenging.

"When my firstborn turned a year old, everything changed. Before she began walking, I knew I could get some rest because I could always keep an eye on her. No more of that after walking was mastered. Lola was incredibly active, and all the weight I gained by being in the house that first year came off in weeks. I was constantly running right behind her and it was really exhausting.

PARDOXICAL REACTIONS TO CAFFEINE

"My daughter Sharon was only two years old when I discovered that she had drunk an entire cup of my coffee (with cream) while I was using the bathroom. She then took her first ever two-hour nap that day—as opposed to her usual two or three fifteen-minute cat naps a day.

"I was really afraid I had put her into a coma—and all because I hadn't moved my coffee cup out of her reach. But she was fine." After this incident, Marie, 32, a mother with ADD, decided that using caffeine as a sleep-inducer for Sharon (who probably also has ADD, based on her reaction to caffeine) once in awhile was okay.

Is she right? There are no clinical studies stating that children or adults with ADD have a paradoxical reaction to caffeine—that it puts them to sleep. There are many anecdotal reports that it has this effect, but we just don't know for sure.

Jenny says, "Now I know about my ADD and how it affected taking care of my kids when they were small, I have lots of advice to impart to other moms! First, get babysitting help, whether you're a stay-at-home mom as I was or you work full time. Not just a few Saturday nights a month to go out with your spouse—although those are important too! But you also need down time during the week too—carve out that time for yourself.

"It's really important to find outside activities so your whole life isn't totally engaged in daily struggles of child rearing and maybe work too. It may sound selfish, but giving yourself time on a regular basis, to do whatever you want to do, whether lolling in a bathtub or biking in the park or something else—is a form of self-preservation. It's sort of like on the airplane when they tell mothers to put the oxygen masks on themselves first in the event of a crash, so they'll be conscious and can help their babies."

A TOTALLY SIMPLE POTTY TRAINING CHART FOR MOMS WITH ADD

Most moms with ADD find it very difficult to use charts on which you are supposed to track points your children earn for good behavior. I can't do them! However, there is one—and only one—chart I have been able to use in parenting my three children. Since it worked well for me pre-ADD diagnosis, it must be a good idea.

1. Buy gold stars that stick on paper. They come in little boxes with about a gazillion of them in each box. One box is enough!

2. Get a piece of paper and write the name of your child (who is at least 2½ years old) in large block letters on top. Show the child the name and admire it.

3. Draw five blocks/rectangles large enough to stick a star inside each.

4. Announce to the child that every time she or he uses the toilet (which you will check on yourself), a gold star will be placed in a block.

5. Explain that after the child has received five gold stars, she will be rewarded with a trip to McDonald's, a visit to the park, or something comparable. A nice reward but not a huge one. It must be a reward that the *child* would like.

6. Put the chart on the refrigerator. Make a big deal out of it.

7. Ignore all potty "accidents" other than cleaning them up.

8. When the child does go potty, act like he won the Academy Award for Best Actor or the Nobel Peace Prize. What a big girl/boy! What a wonderful child! Take her to the refrigerator where she can watch you put the gold star in the block, with great ceremony. Tell your child there are only four more (or three, etc.) to go before the prize is won.

9. If he wasn't there when it happened, when your spouse or significant other comes home, be excited all over again about the successful potty incident. Praise the child extravagantly. Hug the child and beam at her or him. Your partner should do the same.

10. When the child earns that fifth gold star, give her the prize. It doesn't matter how awful behavior was in other things. Nothing can take away a gold star, and the prize is always won if you get the fifth one. Do *not* give it to her beforehand, no matter what. It must be totally earned. If she never earns the fifth gold star, she is probably not ready to be potty trained. Try again in a few months.

"Most of all," adds Jenny, "enlist the help of your spouse. When you feel like you're about to blow, give him a signal to take over so you can remove yourself from the situation in order to recover."

▶ **LIMITS—WITH LOVE**

Can you set limits for a toddler or preschool child? You can—and you should! Don't touch the stove, don't stick your face in the toilet, don't eat ants—all sorts of things little kids might try. You can also teach limits to the child, but not by reasoning with the child, as many parents erroneously think is a good idea. Did you ever see a grown man or woman try to explain to an upset three-year-old why it is morally wrong to bite another child? You stop the behavior, and skip the lecture. It is not age-appropriate.

Instead, provide your child with choices that lead to good behavior. Reward good behavior, whether it occurs by accident or design.

Disciplining Small Children Can Be Difficult for Moms

Many mothers worry about when and how to discipline their children, and moms with ADD worry about this issue more than most. Many experience difficulty with discipline because of their problems with inattentiveness, impatience and so forth. But the mom with ADD who uses the ADD assets she has—of creativity, curiosity, spontaneity, and a sense of humor—can usually come up with a good plan.

For example, often a child can be surprised out of bad behavior by a mom who says or does something startling. Ellie, 34, once stood on her head in the middle of a full-fledged temper tantrum her child was throwing. She isn't quite sure why she did it—but the headstand instantly captivated the child's attention and distracted her from her anger.

If anyone is good at distractions, it's the mom with ADD! Of course you may not wish to stand on your head. You could say something silly or start singing a silly song. Keep in mind that sometimes children misbehave because they are ill, or they are "coming down" with something. If distraction is ineffective, then consider also that the child could be sick or overtired.

Realize that discipline, and many other aspects of parenting, should depend on the child's developmental level of understanding.

Forms of Discipline

There are a variety of ways to discipline children. What's really important—and often very difficult for the mom with ADD—is to be *consistent*. If you tell the child that if she slams her doll down one more time, she is going to be sent to her room, then send her to her room when she slams the doll down again. Don't suddenly decide it would be better to now give her choices of one option or another or, much worse, do nothing at all. Children are constantly "testing" parents, and what they need and want are parents who are reliable in their disciplinary methods.

It's also important for other adults living in your house to be consistent with the discipline you decide upon. If you say that under no circumstances can X be done, but a child knows Dad will always let him do it, then you have a problem. Make sure that you and other adults have worked this issue out.

Here are the key disciplinary techniques most people use:

- Offering choices
- Using time-outs
- Rewarding good behavior, ignoring bad behavior
- Withholding privileges
- Spanking
- Using charts or point systems

Offering Choices

Even small children like the idea that they can choose to do one thing or another. They don't usually stop to think that you are in control of what the choices are. Here are some examples of choices you can give a small child:

- Would you like to stop throwing food now or take a nap?
- Will you stop biting or shall we go home now?

Again, be sure to follow through. If four-year-old Susie keeps throwing her food on the floor, then she has to take the nap. If five-year-old Tommy bites again, you leave. No discussion. To help yourself be consistent, make sure the choices are workable for the child *and* you. If you don't want to (or can't) go home, don't offer it as an option.

The impulsive mom with ADD may suddenly announce the punishment and then realize it's not fair or workable. I vaguely remember a line from the movie *Hairspray*, in which a teenage girl's parents are so angry with her that they say she is "grounded forever. Even after you are dead!" It was a funny line, in context. But make your punishments more reasonable.

If you have a problem with patience and impulsivity, when your child misbehaves, try counting to ten before you announce the punishment. Then take a deep breath and think about it. Write it down and look at it. Still okay? Go ahead.

Here is an example of choices you can offer a child at age four or five:

- You can say I'm sorry to Susie for knocking down her bridge, *or* you can take a time-out.
- You can pick up your toys now and I'll read you a story, *or* you can go to bed and I'll use the book time to pick up your toys for you.

If you want to use the distraction tactic to counter misbehavior, you could offer silly choices, such as, would you like to fly to the moon or visit the bottom of the ocean? Would you rather be a cow or a rhinoceros?

Using Time-outs

A sort of variation from being told to "stand in the corner," a time-out, or cessation of activities, can be effective sometimes when choices don't work. It's a tactic best used on children aged of 3–6 years. Time-outs can be hard for the mom with ADD, especially if you are distractible or hyperactive. Keep in mind that your job as a parent is to give children what they need, which may not be the same as what they want. Sometimes they "need" time-outs.

You can use a time-out on a bright child as young as 18 months, but one minute is usually enough and only for infractions such as taking another child's toy. Usually distracting a child this young or removing him to another activity is sufficient.

The time-out should not be to an interesting place like the child's room, but instead should be someplace boring—a chair in the kitchen or sitting on the stairs. Keep the time-outs very brief, no longer than 15 minutes, as a punishment (unless the child violates the time-out, in which case you add more time).

If the child moves before the time-out is over, calmly say, "Every minute out of time-out is another minute added. You are now at sixteen minutes." Do *not* physically restrain the child.

If the tactic of adding time doesn't work and the child jumps up anyway, you make comments such as "I'm sorry we will be spending all day on time-out. We won't have time to _____ (go outside, clean the kitchen). But that's okay because I'll have more time to (do the laundry, read a book). In addition, while all this is going on, the parent needs to continue doing something else rather than paying attention to the child (straighten the pillows, clean the stove, etc.). It doesn't work if you devote 100 percent of your attention to the child, because then he will have no incentive to comply with the time-out.

If the child runs out of the room, pick her up and put her back in the room. Sometimes this can be a frustrating exercise, especially when you and the child both have ADD. Despite this, don't lock the child in the room, because that could be frightening or even dangerous.

Catch Them in the Act of Accidentally Being Good

Another form of discipline is to "catch" your child behaving the way you like and then providing positive reinforcement. When my older children were little (ages 3 and 4), they were good most of the time. But whenever I answered the phone, for some reason, they became cranky and irritable and behaved very badly. I didn't know how to solve this problem because sometimes I had to take short calls. One day, my children were playing quietly in the living room and for some reason, hadn't noticed that the phone had rung and I was talking to someone. So here's what I did.

After the conversation ended, I walked up to the children and praised them lavishly for what *good* children they were and how pleased I was that they were such big children that they could be quiet when Mommy was on the phone. I hugged them both and took them out to play with me in the backyard.

The next time the phone rang, the children were quiet. I praised them again, much less lavishly. After that, I had no problems unless they really needed something urgently. Positive reinforcement—catching someone in the act of behaving the way you want him or her to act—can be very powerful.

You may well say, my children are always acting up; they are never quiet. And, because of your inattentiveness, you are less likely to notice those times when the children are good. But they happen. Even the most hyperactive child on the planet has at least a few nanoseconds when he sits still or behaves in the way that you want. If you work at it, you can catch him in the act. Do remember, however, that we can't expect our children to be serene little angels all the time. Part of being a child is being noisy, messy, and "acting like a baby."

Withholding Privileges

Use this form of discipline only as a last resort, and for purposefully bad behavior. In general, providing choices or using time-outs or catching the child in the act of being good are much better methods of discipline, especially for a small child. But your three-year-old may have trouble imagining beyond a half hour from now if she too has ADD.

Thus, if you tell the a four-year-old child on Monday that she can't go to the movies on Saturday because of her misbehavior, the punishment is far too distant from the "crime." Also, withholding of privileges can be very upsetting if the child's behavior was accidental. For example, breaking a toy is not a bad thing unless it belongs to someone else. When the child breaks her toy, she suffers because she doesn't have the toy anymore. But be sure neither you nor your spouse runs out to replace the toy!

Withholding privileges or toys can be really hard for the mom with ADD, because you may feel guilty or upset about it. If you feel a little inadequate about mothering, a sobbing child can break down your resistance fast. Be sympathetic and understanding. And take the toy away too.

Spanking

Although corporal punishment is legal in nearly all states, most experts believe that it is ineffective at its most benign and abusive at its worst. Corporal punishment involves physical punishments such as spanking, hitting, or slapping. The problem with such punishment, beyond the fact that it doesn't work well, is that often the parent can find her anger escalating as she strikes the child. Another problem is that it teaches the child that it's okay to inflict physical pain on another person.

That said, many people were subjected to mild corporal punishment as children, and most of us are fully functional adults. However, our parents were not told that corporal punishment could be problematic and were encouraged to use it. Today, most experts strongly discourage the use of corporal punishment and most parents realize this.

Realize also that in our own childhoods, many of our mothers were homemakers and we received a lot more praising and positive interactions day in and day out to balance the spankings. Now, with many children in childcare much of the time, parents may have many fewer of the positive episodes to balance out the same number of spankings.

What if you get into a temper yourself and impulsively whack your child on the behind? Will he be emotionally scarred for life? Very doubtful. But it's a good idea for you to find ways to keep that anger under control. Realize that children will misbehave, and if you plan ahead to deal with those incidents, you will be less likely to "lose it."

WORKING WITH YOUR CHILDCARE CENTER ON DISCIPLINE

If your child spends any time in a childcare center, enlist its help with discipline. The staff should be using the same general methods as you are. In fact, sometimes you can try their method if you find that your own disciplinary tactics aren't working.

Using Charts or Point Systems

Many women have been assured that if they try the latest system using charts and awarding points for good behavior, their discipline problems will be solved. What the chart-lovers fail to take into account is that many moms have ADD *themselves*. If you have a hard time remembering things and tend to be distractible, impulsive, and procrastinate, how well do you think a chart system can work, even a very simple one?

My guess is maybe a few weeks, at best. In the previous section, Babies/Toddlers, I described a potty training program using stars and then rewards as incentives. This system worked quickly for me in potty training my three children; however, I strongly suspect that if it had taken more than three weeks, I would have given up on it altogether. The key to my success was that the children were developmentally ready to be trained, and they wanted to be trained. I feel I just gave them a little boost toward success.

Does this mean you should never try a chart system? Paradoxically, I will say no. A chart may work for you and it may not. The only way to know is to try it. If it doesn't work, don't immerse yourself in guilt and self-blame. Just realize that it didn't work for you. Maybe another, simpler system would work. Or maybe formalized behavioral charts are not for you. You can only know for sure by trying.

SELF-DOUBTS CAN BE VERY DESTRUCTIVE

"Before I knew I had ADD, I blamed myself horribly," said Fran, 39, mother of two. "I'd wanted children desperately and when they arrived, I felt like I was the worst mother because I couldn't handle the crying, the whining, the tugging, and the constant neediness that's involved in raising children.

"As they got older, other negative self-talk nagged at me. Why couldn't I keep up with all the papers that needed signing? Why was I unable to bake brownies for every school occasion, like the other moms did? Why did I hate volunteering at school? What was wrong with me?

"Here's what I learned: We *must* remember that we are wired differently from non-ADD adults. We have to forgive ourselves for not being "perfect parents," whatever that actually means."

▶ YOUR OWN EXPECTATIONS AS A NEW MOM

Before you bring your baby home or when she's still an infant, it's a good idea to start thinking about what you believe raising children will be like. You may have realistic expectations for yourself, or you may be an incredible taskmaster. You may also have some unrealistic ideas of children. To find out some of your views about children, take this short self-test, answering true or false to each statement:

	True	False
1. If my children act up, I am a bad mother.		
2. If my children act up, other people think I am a bad mother.		
3. If my preschool child is angry with me, that means I have done something wrong.		
4. I should try to find ways to help my child *not* have ADD like me.		
5. Other mothers have secret knowledge on how to be good parents. I don't and wonder why they do.		
6. If I get angry with my four-year-old, this means there's something wrong with me.		
7. If my child seems generally unhappy or distressed, it must mean I don't love her enough.		
8. If I make a mistake, such as yelling at my child, he will be traumatized for life.		

Let's take a brief look at your responses. If you answered "true" to question 1 (if your children act up, then you are a bad mother), in most cases, you have been misled. Children misbehave sometimes even when mothers are extremely good parents. This is a fact of life. If your child is constantly misbehaving, a good mother will find out if the child is ill, or has a problem, or if she should reconsider her form of discipline. Sometimes a therapist is a good idea in such a case.

If you answered "true" to question 2 (if your children act up, other people will think you are a bad mother), you are partially right. There are plenty of judgmental people, willing and eager to put down parents for their children's behavior. There are also plenty of understanding and supportive people out there too.

What about question 3 (if your preschool child is angry with you)? Does that mean you have done something wrong? Possibly. But it's also possible that your child is angry because she really doesn't feel like putting away her toys, taking a nap, and so forth. You need to evaluate the situation in the context of what is going on, not only from her frame of reference but your own. It's hard enough to sort out your own feelings, but you also need to attempt to sort out what your children are thinking and feeling as well.

Some therapists say that mothers have asked them how they can make their children *not* have ADD, and you may have wondered about this yourself, which was the purpose for question 4. The answer is easy: You can't. You can help your child who has ADD, but you can't magically make it go away.

Question 5 addressed a common myth: That other people, especially women who don't have ADD, have special inborn knowledge of how to be a good parent. Although it's true that some women seem more capable of caring for children than others, the fact is other new mothers don't know much more than you do. If they do, they learned it the hard way, by asking questions and reading books and by learning through trial and error.

Question 6 addressed a very common fear among many mothers, whether they have ADD or not: If you become angry with your child, then you are bad. Realistically, sometimes your child will annoy you and your anger will be quite natural. If you strike out at the child or punish him severely for a minor infraction, or if you berate him for long periods of time—these are all examples of anger run amok. They may also be examples of underlying psychological problems. Taken to extremes, such behaviors are abusive. Anger in and of itself is not abusive. It is merely a human emotion. What's important is what you *do* with that anger.

Question 7 indicates the egocentricity with which many mothers may view the world. If your child is unhappy, it's your fault. Is it also your fault if it rains or snows? Of course, sometimes your child may be distressed by something you did. Again, consider the context of what has happened, from both your viewpoint and your child's.

Another common notion, reflected in question 8, is that if you make an error in judgement and, for example, start screaming at your child, then he will be scarred for life. Certainly nobody likes to be shrieked at. But children are far more adaptable than was once believed. If you apologize to the child (and yes, it is okay for an adult to apologize), and avoid any more screaming fits, all should be well in most cases.

In this chapter, I presented advice for the mom with ADD who is parenting an infant or toddler, and offered advice on basic discipline. A self-test to help you think about your realistic and unrealistic ideas about parenting was also included.

8

Parenting the School-Age Child: The Basics

**Mothers are expected to organize the daily liv-
ing activities of the whole family, to keep a neat
house, and to have dinner on the table every
night. We're also supposed to be interested in
kids' activities even when they can be incredibly
boring, like board games. And, on top of that,
we're expected to be active in our kids' schools.
I mean, who can remember to bring brownies—
let alone make them?**
—Denise, 35, mother of two school-age children

This chapter offers helpful advice for the mother of a school-age child, including:

- Realities of parents
- Organizational nightmares
- Two-way interactions: children affect parents too
- Common childhood ploys to watch out for
- Rules that you can stick to

▶ REALITIES OF PARENTING

If you think that parenting a child of any age always should be like an idyllic
mother-and-child scene from a holiday card, you will be very disappointed. But if
you realize that there are bad times and good times, you'll be much better prepared
and able to cope more effectively as a parent.

ARE ADOPTED CHILDREN MORE PRONE TO ADD?

Some studies of clinical populations (children receiving therapy) indicate a higher than expected rate of adopted children with ADD, although estimates vary greatly on the level of risk. Many hypotheses have been devised to explain why adopted children may be at greater risk for ADD, ranging from the impulsive behavior of their biological parents (with regard to unplanned pregnancies) to the anxiety a birth mother may have transferred to the fetus in utero and other theories.

There are also those who say that adoptive parents are more likely to take their children to a therapist when the child needs help. This tendency could be combined with the risk factors described earlier.

A high genetic linkage has been demonstrated between adults and their biological children (whether adopted or not) who have ADD. The birth mother or birth father of an adopted child may have exhibited the key symptoms of ADD, including high levels of distractibility, impulsivity, and other common characteristics.

An adopted child may have a higher risk of ADD than children who were not adopted. That risk seems to be more genetic than environmental. Mothers should provide the love and assistance their children, adopted or not, with ADD need.

The following truths may be hard for any mother, but may be especially hard for some of us ADD moms to learn and accept. Some of us are perfectionistic or idealistic, and many of us are extremely hard on ourselves. If our child is unhappy, it's often our first impulse to wonder what it was that *we* did wrong. Of course, it's good to consider your own behavior and to change it when needed. But the problem doesn't always stem from you.

The following paragraphs deal with some basic hard truths about parenting.

1. **Sometimes your child won't like you.** If you want to always be loved *and* liked by your child, this is very normal. But if you really expect it to happen, think again! Sometimes you will have to make decisions that your child won't like, and you will be the "bad guy"—this is part of being a parent. Not a fun part, but a quite necessary part. This can be hard for the mom with ADD to accept, because she may have spent years—or most of her life—trying to please others and make things be all right.

2. **Sometimes you won't like your child.** Horrors! Maybe your child won't like you, okay, but you will always and forever like your child, won't you? If not, aren't you the proverbial "bad mother?" Note that I am not saying you won't *love* your child. I believe we should give our children unconditional love, and that they should know that no matter what, we will still love them. This does not mean we have to approve of their behavior, and that in turn means sometimes a child is so annoying and obnoxious that we just don't like him or her on that day. The liking part nearly always comes back, because eventually the child behaves in a positive way again. The love part underlies all and never changes.

3. Sometimes you'll make mistakes. Nobody likes to make mistakes, but we make them anyway, such as not letting a child do something that we probably should have allowed or permitting an activity that was beyond her age. We made an error in judgment. We are not evil people who should be condemned for all time. But we made a mistake. The important thing about mistakes is that they can teach you so much. As long as you learn something, and, when applicable, apologize to your child, mistakes are usually not so horrible.

4. Sometimes you will embarrass your child. Sometimes your silly behavior may embarrass your child. Sometimes your mere existence will embarrass your child, particularly after the child is about age 12. It doesn't matter how great you look—that is irrelevant. For children at certain ages, mothers are inherently embarrassing. There's nothing that you can do about it but accept that this, too, will pass.

5. Sometimes your child will embarrass you. Here is another given: Your child will embarrass you. You might assume that after you've lain in a hospital bed having your baby, spread-eagled and fully exposed, with all sorts of people running in and out of the room, you could never be embarrassed again.

You are wrong. Starting before school and through adolescence (and sometimes beyond), there will be times when they embarrass you. They'll repeat things that you said to others, they'll behave obnoxiously, they'll do all sorts of things. Mostly, they don't mean to embarrass you; but once in awhile, they do mean it.

6. Sometimes your child's behavior mirrors yours. Do you think it would be great to have a clone of yourself? I don't. That person would have all your good predispositions—and the bad ones too. Your children aren't clones of you, but they will often imitate your behavior, whether consciously or unconsciously. And sometimes you won't like it. You may not even be sure whether it's behavior meant to annoy you.

SIMPLE MORNING MEDICINE TIP

If your sleepy school-age child needs medication in the morning, and you find yourself struggling to get her to wake up and take it, try this. Get a plastic or paper cup of water and tell the child to hold it as you hand it to her. In most cases, the child will wake up enough so that he won't spill it on himself. You can then hand him the medicine. You may have to allow the child to spill the water on himself once before it makes an impression. In that case, say, "Oh dear, you spilled the water, let me get you more."

Do not yell at the child for spilling, and do not accept blame for what happened. Just get him more water (and maybe some dry clothes too). Give him another cup of water and then his medicine.

For example, if you have a habit of twirling your hair, and one day, you notice your daughter doing the same thing, you might grit your teeth and think that she is making fun of you. But is she? Maybe. But maybe not. It's possible that she may have a habit similar to yours, and that habit could be as hardwired in her as it is in you.

7. **Sometimes no matter what you do, you can't help.** I think this is the toughest lesson to learn: Sometimes we can't fix things, no matter how much we want to. Our children are in physical or emotional pain, and other people have to be trusted to solve the problem. This doesn't mean that we don't continue trying. But it may well mean that we have to stop beating ourselves up mentally about how we have "failed" our child because we can't resolve a difficult situation in her favor.

▶ **ORGANIZATIONAL NIGHTMARES**

It's hard to be sufficiently organized when your child is an infant or preschooler. But guess what! Things get tougher. One of the biggest problems for the ADD mom is keeping track of reams of paper that accompany a school-age child.

Laurie, 31, describes quite bluntly what life was like for her when her children were little, and what she has learned since then.

"When they are babies, you could buy a ton of cute little containers of baby food and crates of formula. Close your eyes and pick a jar. But school age? That means . . . cooking! Decisions! Planning! If you have a kid who only eats peanut butter and jelly every day, you're in luck. In my case, neither of my kids will eat sandwiches. Figuring out what to feed them has been a nightmare."

GETTING BLAMED FOR NO MITTENS

"If a child doesn't have a hat, scarf or mittens in the winter, it's looked upon as the mother's fault—'I can't believe she'd let her kid go out like that.' It's hard when you get blamed for forgetting things your kids need," said Alice, 35, mother of one.

Some ideas Alice could try, using the creative aspect of her ADD:

- Put mitten clips on the mitten and coat so they're always there.
- Leave extra mittens/hat/scarf (with his name on it) in child's desk at school or in the pocket of his backpack.
- Put a big box of mittens by the front door or where you hang up coats, so the child sees them as he is getting dressed to go out.

Laurie continued, "Along with meal-planning issues come the billions of papers that kids bring home from school, homework, forms to fill out, and other paper-related activities. An ADD nightmare. Also, by school age, there's a good chance you have another child or two, or three. Juggling all the children's needs is quite a daunting task. Let's not even discuss laundry, after-school lessons, haircuts, and clothes buying.

"What I found difficult too, was teaching my kids to be neat and organized when I was having problems in those areas. It really was the blind leading the blind. What to do? Lower your expectations of what you can do as a mom. It doesn't make you any *less* of a mom. Think about your strengths. And if keeping a sock drawer tidy isn't one of them, force yourself to let that go. It's just not worth it."

Laurie thinks that raising older children can be as challenging as raising little ones and urges time off for mom. Can't afford it? Try trading a good or service. For example, if you're great at the computer, offer to show your baffled pal how to use the Internet in exchange for some babysitting time.

Don't forget to ask your husband or significant other to help out with responsibilities, such as packing the school lunches and driving the kids places.

LIKE A KID IN A CANDY STORE

Avoid taking your children grocery shopping if you can. Ask a friend or neighbor to watch them. It's too easy to be distracted and to end up buying things you don't want or need—while forgetting important items.

▶ IT'S A TWO-WAY INTERACTION: CHILDREN AFFECT PARENTS TOO

I read somewhere for a mom with ADD, having children is like having a freight train running through your head!
—Maureen, 40, mother of two

It's very common for parents to think that only children are affected by our actions, and somehow we deflect the impact of their behavior on *us*. This is a silly view held by some social scientists, as well as people in society, who assume if children misbehave, it's invariably their mothers' fault.

For example, in one study of hyperactive boys, researchers noticed mothers behaved in a very negative way. They yelled a lot and were constantly reminding their sons to do this and that. They never seemed to let up. Those poor boys; their mothers were making them crazy.

Then a funny thing happened. The hyperactive boys were medicated and their behavior improved drastically. But the behavior of the "mean" mothers changed as well. The moms stopped yelling and ended constant reminders. Light bulb! It occurred to some researchers that the reason why the mothers had been yelling before and constantly reminding before was in *reaction* to the behavior of their sons. Sure, constant yelling isn't a good thing; but it was apparently not the cause of the boys' behavior. Instead, it may have been a reaction to their behavior. When the behavior changed, the mothers adjusted their parenting as well.

As you might imagine, this concept was quite a shock to psychologists, and most of them still don't believe it. After all, we're *adults*. We're in charge. That's the theory anyway. We have the financial power, the parental power, and the moral authority. But we are affected, sometimes quite profoundly, by our children's behavior.

Does this mean, then, that we parents have *no* control? Of course not. As long as we are aware that children can be manipulative; and as long as we realize that children are not saintly, pure creatures but immature people reacting to their own minds, to their peers, and to *us*, their parents, we will be a lot better off. There are three basic principles you need to remember:

1. **We affect our children to varying degrees.** The greatest impact occurs during infancy and toddlerhood.

2. **Our children's behavior affects us even during infancy and toddlerhood.** The colicky baby is more difficult than the quiet child.

3. **Most children use ploys to convince their parents to give them what they want.** This is not evil or immoral. It is, for the most part, very common. You did it too.

We Affect Our Children to Varying Degrees

When our children are infants and toddlers, we have a great deal of control over them, including what they eat, whom they play with, and so forth. Even when they go to a childcare center, it's one we chose. If we don't like it, we put them in another place. After our children leave for school, however, our influence wanes. It continues to fade as a child grows and her peers become much more important. In her book, *The Nurture Assumption: Why Children Turn Out the Way They Do,* Judith Rich Harris argues that peers have a dramatic influence on children of all ages, including preschoolers.

Our Children's Behavior Affects Us in Varying Degrees

It's not only your child who is cranky and unreasonable, and who might throw a temper tantrum when he is ill or overtired. Adults do this too. You had a terrible day at work and you didn't get enough sleep. Maybe you were hyperfocusing on a work project and forgot to eat lunch. You get home and you're upset and exhausted. And your child starts asking for this or that. Maybe her behavior isn't that bad. But you explode anyway.

Wait a minute. Isn't this section supposed to be about how our children affect us, not our own behavior? Yes, it is, and the child did affect the mom in this case, through no grievous fault of the child. She was a little whiney and that's all Mom could take. In another situation, when Mom was not upset and overtired, she could deal with the normal petulance that children can exhibit.

The point is, parents are affected in varying degrees by their children, depending on their own inner states *as well as* the children's behavior.

Common Childhood Ploys

Some children with ADD have what author H. Joseph Horacek calls "brainstorms." The fury is massive, but when it is over, the child has forgotten about it. Like a sudden thunderstorm in the summer, the sun comes out and everything is okay again—from the child's perspective. She may be bewildered about why Mom or Dad is so annoyed with her.

Another issue that I think is important to mention are all the little ploys that children use to get what they want—because so often, they work! In fact, they are especially effective when used on a guilt-stricken mom with ADD. So don't fall for any of the following.

Everybody/Nobody Does That

If you don't think you used this tactic when you were a child, you probably either forgot about using it or you were a very unusual child. Many children tell their parents that they should receive a certain item or be allowed to have a certain privilege because everybody else can have it or do it. Or nobody else has to be restricted, as you are restricting your child. In most cases, the child isn't correct. Other children aren't allowed to have or do what he wants. But it really doesn't matter, because you need to act in the best interests of your own child.

ANGER MANAGEMENT

What can children do about anger and frustration? Experts say it's good for parents to help children learn effective ways of "letting off steam." One good tactic is active exercise: bicycling, running long distance, and playing games like soccer or basketball.

They can also learn other techniques used by adults with ADD, such as giving themselves a time-out to leave the area that contains a person they're angry with. Or recalling a pleasant, calm scene in their lives and fixating on that until they calm down sufficiently.

Your child may be right that other children are allowed to do things he can't. Every other child may be allowed to watch vicious programs on television—and every other parent may be wrong.

There are also cases where it is possible that you are being restrictive. If you are making your 10-year-old child go to bed at 7:30 at night, it probably is too early. If your child says that you are treating her like a baby, maybe you are.

Evaluate your own actions and decide if they are reasonable in the light of what is reasonable for most children your child's age. If you aren't sure, obtain parenting books that talk about developmental stages. Ask your pediatrician. Talk to other parents. Then make your own decision.

I Can't Find It

This ploy can work very well sometimes on a mom with ADD, primarily because *she* is prone to losing things. However, your child may tell you that she can't find something for any and all of the following reasons:

- She hasn't looked for the item.
- She doesn't want you to see the item (for example, a paper with a bad grade).
- She looked for it, but only briefly. Another search could turn the item up.

If you think it's remotely possible that your child is playing any of these mind games with you, the following responses from you might generate the desired action—of having your child look for the missing thing.

- I'll look for it in your room—and while I'm in there, I'll just pick up a little bit. (Many children over age 8 don't want you to go in their room and see the chaos.)
- I'll give you another chance to look for it, and then after you find it we can _____ (fill in the blank with something fun that the child likes.)
- Maybe I should call your teacher. (If the missing item is a school paper and has a bad grade on it, the last thing your child will want is for you to call her teacher.)
- I know! I'll have Jimmy see if he can find it in your room! (Most siblings don't like their other sibs to go through their stuff.)

It's Too Hard for Me

I think that moms with ADD have more compassion for all children. What they don't understand, they go find out about instead of looking down at the child. We get on the floor, up the tree, and down in the mud, whatever it takes.
—Lucy, 32, mother of one child

It's almost an innate kind of "programming" for mothers to want to help their children and make their lives easier. But the problem is that you can overdo that and unknowingly make your child overly dependent on you. The job of a good parent is to love and care for her children, but at the same time, help them gain the skills so they can grow up to be effective adults. We give them "roots" and we give them "wings"—and that is one of the hard parts of parenthood.

As she listens to her child say that a task is too hard, it's very easy for a mom with ADD to remember how tough life was for her when *she* was a child, and nobody understood she really was trying her best—even though some people kept insisting that she was not. Consider the context of the situation. Your child may have similar problems, but she is not you. When your child says, "It's too hard for me, Mommy," brake your impulsive desire to rush in and "make it better." Maybe it is too hard. But maybe not.

Sometimes children experience insults and upsets, and that is part of growing up. One of the difficult tasks for the mom with ADD is distinguishing between what a child can do and what is genuinely too hard. One way to find out is to let the child perform a task and allow him to fail—or succeed.

You're Mean

Who wants to be a mean, nasty mother? The mom with ADD wants to be a good mom, but needs to realize that just because kids are unhappy with her does *not* mean that she is doing the wrong thing. I recall long ago when my older son, then age nine, wanted me to drop him off at a new friend's house. I drove there and it was in a very bad neighborhood, with many tough-looking characters hanging about. I told him to forget it, we were going home.

He was furious with me and said I was snobby, mean, awful, and so forth; but I would not back down. A few days later my son apologized to me. Another friend's mother *had* dropped him off at that trailer in the bad neighborhood. He told my son he was terrified the whole time, and the boy's father was drunk and yelling and screaming. You can bet that made me feel happy that I had stuck to my guns!

It's Your Fault/Not My Fault

Another ploy that is too easy for moms with ADD to believe is "it's your fault." Many of us are so programmed to accept self-blame, after hearing throughout much of our childhood and adulthood that we should "try harder" and "if only" we would remember to do such and such, everything would be okay.

If you don't fall for the "Mom's fault" ploy, a corollary that may follow is that whatever the problem, it's not really your child's fault. Overprotective moms are particularly prone to falling for the "it's not my fault" excuse. Rather than arguing fault, it's best to shape behavior by offering children choices when possible and teaching them to accept consequences for their actions.

GOOD COMMUNICATION IS A TWO-WAY STREET

Are you following these simple communication rules?

- Don't talk through or beyond your child. Instead, look directly at him or her. If you need to communicate something important, get down to the child's eye level.

- Is your child looking at you as you speak? Not an unswerving gaze but at least paying some attention?

- Are you conveying one or two main messages? One at a time is better.

- Are you seeking feedback? Don't ask questions that can be answered with yes or no, such as, "Did you hear me?" Ask the child to summarize what you said.

- Are you listening to the child's response even if it's not what you want to hear?

- Are you watching the child's body language for emotional responses?

- Are you concluding your remarks with your own summary of what is important?

- Are you using a tone of voice you would want to hear yourself?

- Instead of yelling, try speaking *softer* as a listening inducement. It may sound crazy but it can work well. Be sure to say the child's name first, in a loud enough voice, and then "turn down the volume" for the rest of your message.

▶ CREATE RULES AND STICK WITH THEM

Most experts agree that it's really important for parents to be consistent in their rules for children. If you tell your child she can never ever play outside your fenced yard without permission, but sometimes you yell at her when she tests you and sometimes you don't, this lack of consistency is very confusing for children. It's also confusing if Mom says something is not okay but Dad says, sure, go ahead. Avoid these common problems!

And yet, the mom with ADD may think that it's easier to just let the child go ahead and do the thing she's not supposed to do—is it really that bad? The point is, if the rule wasn't important, then why did Mom make it in the first place? Rules should be flexible as children grow in maturity and the capability to deal with the world. But "flexible" doesn't mean it's not okay today but then it's okay tomorrow.

A Self-Test on Rules

Ask yourself the following questions, answering yes or no to each one.

	Yes	No
1. My spouse or significant other and I use the same forms of discipline.		
2. My children know when they must come in at night.		
3. My children know when they must ask permission.		
4. If my children break one of my rules, I don't let it go unless the child is ill or there is a very good reason.		
5. My family's basic rules are written down and posted in a place where everyone can see them.		

Did you answer yes to most of these questions? If so, you are consistent in your discipline. If not, find ways to be more consistent, whether it's written reminders, asking your spouse to let you know when you slip up (privately), or other means.

Writing the Rules Down and Posting Them

Many experts believe that it's important to write down the rules and post them in a place where everyone can see them. If you do this, I recommend that you keep the rules very simple and don't make too many of them. Here are some examples of possible rules:

- The last one in the house has to lock up (for children over age 10).
- If you break something, clean it up unless it's too dangerous. In that case, tell Mom or Dad.
- Turn the television, record player, radio, computer, or any other devices off before you leave the house.
- Put your dirty clothes in _____ (wherever you want them to put their dirty clothes).

When your child starts kindergarten, everything changes. Peers and teachers become very important to your child. In this chapter, I covered the realities of parenting a school-age child and explained that adults affect children, but children themselves affect their parents in many ways. One way is by using common childhood ploys, such as "everybody else can do this," "it's too hard," and others. The mom with ADD may be more prone to buy into these childhood ploys and needs to keep on her parenting toes.

9

The ADD Mom and the Adolescent: Now *There* Is a Challenge!

No, you may not cryogenically freeze your teenagers into suspended animation and have them thawed out at age 21—as appealing as that idea may seem sometimes to the parent of an adolescent. Instead, you must learn how to cope with the hormonal storms and the breaking away from you as your child struggles toward adulthood.

Of course, it isn't all bad; there are plenty of fun times. But the fact is sometimes adolescence will remind you of when your child was two and his favorite word was "No!" This chapter offers advice to the ADD mom parenting an adolescent, including:

- Recognizing adolescent angst vs. plain old bad behavior
- Considering boundaries and expectations
- Adapting to your teenager's changing needs
- Providing choices within discipline

▶ ADOLESCENT ANGST VS. PLAIN-OLD BAD BEHAVIOR

Most of us think of adolescence as a very difficult time in a person's life—and it often can be. In fact, being an adolescent today is probably much harder than being a teenager when I was growing up—and you may remember it this way too. We had very clear-cut rules that are much hazier today. For example, people weren't supposed to have sex in high school, and they certainly weren't supposed to be making babies. Now such behavior is considered acceptable, if not normal, and their peers consider adolescents who aren't "sexually active" odd.

Freedom is a double-edged sword. When you know what the rules are, even if you don't like them, there is a clear standard. Today, the "rules" are far less clear.

Society still has rules, of course. Adolescents are legally barred from drinking alcohol, and in all states they may not buy cigarettes. But when some adolescents drink or smoke anyway, are people that shocked or distressed? Often they are not.

In some families, parents actually allow their underage children to drink alcohol in their home, reasoning "at least he's doing it here," or "at least he's not driving a car." These parents rationalize their own illegal behavior of providing alcohol to a minor child. It doesn't matter if it is *your* minor or someone else's child: It is still illegal.

GOOD MANIPULATION/BAD MANIPULATION

Teenagers can be very manipulative—but it isn't always bad, as long as you are aware that they are doing it! Here's an example of a "good" manipulation. My husband, the one who helps our son with algebra, was away on a trip. Since Dad wasn't home, my son asked me to help, but I pleaded ignorance to linear equations. I couldn't remember that high school stuff. So my son said, "Mom, you are a very fast learner. I bet you could figure this stuff out in fifteen minutes or less." Then he left the room.

That was a challenge I could not resist. I picked up his math book and read over the examples of how to do the problems. Then I tried a few problems, getting them wrong at first and then figuring them out. My son was not surprised when I called him and said, "Well, okay, maybe I could help you. A little."

Here's an example of "bad" manipulation. "Mom, can I have five dollars so I can go to McDonald's with the neighbors? I promise I'll clean up my room as soon as I get home!" The right answer is usually "no." Why? Because getting promises fulfilled after the teen already had the reward can be very hard. Whenever possible, work first and money (or other reward) second.

Another problem with condoning alcohol consumption by teenagers at your home is that it's tacit approval of all teenage drinking, despite other messages parents think they are sending a child. The health risks of drinking and smoking are quite real.

Drinking isn't cute for teens, and too many children end up dead or maimed for life because of drunken driving. If your child actually experiences a hangover from excessive drinking, I think it's a good idea to be as noisy and obnoxious as possible and hold off on the sympathetic mom part. Others report that loudly saying such things as, "I bet you feel really bad! But it will get better—in a few hours," also works to discipline teens.

What if you know your adolescent is smoking? You actively discourage it, but he somehow obtains cigarettes. Do you allow him to smoke in your home? If you smoke, you are tacitly encouraging your child to smoke; however, you are an adult and he is a minor and you make the rules. Remember, though, that actions speak louder than words. If you really don't want your child to smoke, work on quitting yourself. And if you don't smoke, how could you possibly consider allowing your child to smoke in your home?

Why Is He Mad at You?

Sometimes it doesn't take much to upset a teenager. He may have noticed a few pimples on his face and agonized that he's developing acne. Everyone will be repulsed by his appearance and no girl will look at him, ever. He is sure of this. It doesn't matter if you tell him he's a handsome boy. You're his mother—you are supposed to think this!

Your daughter may have tried out a new hairstyle and received taunts and criticisms from others. It may not seem like much, but when the most important people to you are your peers, it's very important indeed what they think of you.

Since teens usually don't want to scream or cry in front of their friends, you can guess who gets to see the screaming and crying. And if you're a mom with ADD who finds yelling or confusing behavior nearly intolerable, it can be a rough ride.

Keep in mind that your adolescent is really not attempting to inflict psychological torture on you; for example, when he asks you to wash his jeans and you wash the ones that are *not* Levis and he can't possibly wear *those*. Except he forgot to tell you that when he said, "Mom, could you wash my jeans for me?"

If his frustration devolves into verbal abuse, don't put up with it. When a child behaves badly, he needs to suffer the consequences. One consequence for this particular offense could be to tell the teenager you are not doing his laundry for a certain period of time. Or assign extra chores, invoke a loss of privileges, or ground him.

Whenever Possible, Offer Your Adolescent Choices

It's a good idea to offer children of any age a choice, from asking your three-year-old whether she wants the blue ball or the red ball all the way to asking your teenager if he wants to either wash the dishes or mow the lawn before he can take the car. Of course, you can expect him to say he doesn't want to do either one. But you stick to offering choices, and most kids will feel empowered by this option. They will not admit it, but kids like clear rules and options, with no guesswork involved. This means consistency on the part of the mom with ADD, which can be a challenge.

Sometimes offering choices can help you out of a mini-crisis. Carole, 46, mother of an adult daughter and a 12-year-old son, had to go on a two-day trip. She left her daughter in charge, assuring her son that no, this was *not* babysitting. It's just that Tammy was 21 and could drive a car and make decisions—which was why she was in charge. Tammy called Carole the next morning at the hotel and said Evan absolutely refused to take his medicine. Nothing worked. Carole told Tammy to put Evan on the phone.

"She is not babysitting me! I'm not taking my medicine from her!" said Evan. Carole didn't really want Evan dispensing his Ritalin himself, but it was clear that he was firm that Tammy could not give it to him. Suddenly, Carole hit on an idea. "What if Tammy takes the medicine out of the bottle and puts it on the counter and leaves the room. And then you get a glass of water and just take the medicine yourself?" she suggested. "Okay!" said Evan. Problem averted. He still felt like he had some control and wasn't being treated like a "baby"—and that was all he really wanted.

▶ CONSIDERING BOUNDARIES AND EXPECTATIONS

All children want a certain amount of privacy; but in most cases, adolescents are the most eager to preserve their privacy. They don't want you in their rooms, they don't want you looking at their belongings, and they'd prefer that you just leave them alone altogether. Except when they need a ride to the mall or permission to go to a party or on a class trip. Then you are suddenly Ms. Popularity again!

The Open-Door Policy

How much privacy should you give a teenager? This is a tough one: You don't want to be an overbearing mother, and at the same time you'd prefer that there not be any wild sex orgies behind the closed doors of your teens' rooms. So you need to make some basic rules.

It may sound extremely Victorian, but I think it's best to keep the bedroom door open when your teenage child has a friend of the opposite sex in his or her room. In fact, you may take sexual pressure off your child by the knowledge that anyone could walk by anytime and thus he better watch it. This doesn't mean kids won't sexually act out, but it may well mean they don't have sex in their bedrooms—at least, while you're around with that open-door policy intact.

Should the child be allowed to lock his door? If he or she is alone, I don't have a problem with that, although I want to be sure there's a way to enter in case of an emergency. So get a key and put it in a place where it won't be lost.

What about when the child goes out? If the child is worried other siblings will take his things—and his fears are reasonable— it's probably okay to let him lock his room while at school or away somewhere else. But again, you need to have a key yourself.

Should you go into the room when the child is not there? You may need to, to put clothes away or get an item of yours that she took in there. But going into your child's room should not be an excuse to search for evidence of what's going on with her life, and—if she keeps one—you should not read her private journal or diary, except under one circumstance: You have good evidence the child has a problem with depression, drug use, illegal activities, or suicidal or aggressive intent. You don't want the imminent safety of your child or someone else to be threatened.

If your child has ADD, the room may be pretty chaotic looking, even your worst nightmare. It's best to get the child to pick up the room, especially since a teenager is perfectly capable of doing the job. If you see obvious health or safety hazards, or items that someone could trip over in the dark, or a lamp that's turned on, move the skates and shut off the lamp. But leave the rest alone. For most moms with ADD, disorganization is part of our nature and a messy room doesn't bother many of us. For the rest, we dislike the disorganization but may be too distracted to deal with it.

What's Mine Is Mine—and What's Yours Is Mine, Too

Despite the adolescent's strident demands that you leave his or her items alone, the ironic aspect of living with a teenager can also mean that he or she thinks your items are fair game. Or, as the title of this section reads, "What's mine is mine. But what's yours is mine, too." Don't let your adolescent get away with that! Make sure she requests permission before taking your CD player, your clothes, or anything else that is yours.

It's important for the adolescent to respect your boundaries and your privacy and ownership of items too. In a recent cartoon strip called "Zits," the adolescent character Jeremy is wearing his father's shirt without permission. When his father issues a mild challenge, Jeremy retorts, "I thought we were a family. I thought that meant we shared resources willingly and without barriers," and so on. His father let him wear the shirt. Jeremy came back with four other shirts in hand, saying, "Does that go for these too?"

Just because your child can argue effectively and knows how to use emotional manipulation does not mean you should respond to it. In an earlier chapter, I discussed the importance of saying no—and moms with ADD need to learn to use this word a lot.

▶ ADAPTING TO YOUR TEENAGER'S CHANGING NEEDS

The teen years can be hell for a mother with ADD if you don't have a sense of humor.
—Sandy, 43, mother of two teens

As your child becomes an adolescent and grows toward adulthood, you'll need to give him or her more freedom—assuming that he or she can handle it and earn it by obeying rules you set. Of course, you will need to adjust or change your rules. What is appropriate bedtime for a 10-year-old child is not reasonable for a 16-year-old. This does not mean that a 16-year-old should be allowed to stay up all night. Now more than ever it's important to do well in school, and "growing boys and girls" still need their sleep—at least eight hours of it per night. Save the late nights for Friday and Saturday nights, if the child has earned late-night privileges according to the rules you set.

Some mothers use an alternative strategy: They let their children stay up as late as they want to, but they still have to go to school, obtain the best grades they can, and fulfill their home responsibilities too. This may teach them to organize their time better, although it probably is a strategy best used with non-ADD adolescents.

"Because I've now learned how to handle their ADD—and my own—I think that the teen years have been the easiest yet. I'm not as frustrated as I used to be and I am able to talk to my teens and help them deal with ADD in more positive ways. Both my son and daughter have told me they really appreciate that I have given them tools to live their lives," said Adrienne, 45, mother of two teenagers.

Adds Joan, 49, mother of two adolescents, "I have seen many mothers, with ADD and not, who are really frustrated with their teens with ADD. If you don't have a good understanding and haven't developed coping skills by the time the kids are teens, it can really be a struggle. Not hopeless, of course, just harder."

▶ DISCIPLINING YOUR ADOLESCENT: CHOICES ARE IMPORTANT

When your child was little, the choices you offered her were easy. As the mother of an adolescent, you'll find they become harder. Giving your teenager the keys to your car can be pretty terrifying, for two reasons. You don't want your child to have an accident, and you don't want him to wreck your means of transportation either! Obviously, you check him or her out first by driving around with them to make sure they know the basics.

As the parent of a teenager, you need to make some key tough decisions about your policies on the following issues. I'll address some of these issues in this section:

- Dating
- Driving
- Acceptable sexual behavior for teens
- Schoolwork and grades
- Extracurricular activities
- After-school jobs
- Participation in family events
- Participation in religious activities
- Drugs, alcohol, and other illegal behaviors

I suggest that you take this list—and add any items not on it that are important to you—and prioritize it, with "1" being the most important item. Write down what you expect from the child, to help you clarify it in your own mind. If you don't think teenagers should be allowed to date until age 16, then write that down.

Prioritize items that are important to you even if you think your child doesn't have a problem with them. For example, if you are opposed to more than one extracurricular activity, say so, even if your child hasn't joined any clubs or teams to date. If you think it's important for your adolescent to go to the annual family reunion, say so, even though he never protested before now. Situations can change rapidly when you're talking about adolescents. What was okay last week may seem unacceptable this week. And don't assume your child automatically knows what's important to you. Maybe, maybe not.

Create rules for the three or four items most important to you, and negotiate the rules for other items on your list. For example, if the child wants to take an after-school job, and this is low on your list of priorities, you can negotiate with the child how to handle this. You may decide the child can take the job if her grades stay the same, or other conditions are fulfilled.

When you are a mom with ADD, it's best to put these ideas in writing, so you can refer to them later if you need to. A good idea is to type them on the computer and save the file, so you can print it out later if you lose the original printout.

The following sections include some basics on decisions you will need to make about your policies on these various issues. Because you are the best judge of what is right for your child, I won't set any specific parameters for you.

Dating

When your child becomes a teenager, he or she will eventually begin to take interest in dating. Rather than frantically making up your dating policy the day your teen casually mentions she wants to go out with a cute boy she just met, it's a good idea to think it out ahead of time and to discuss it with your teenager.

Here are some decisions you will need to make:

1. **When is it okay for your teen to go out with others in a group dating situation?** It's really up to you to decide when it's okay for boys and girls to go out together with groups of others. You need to take into consideration what is the norm; and if that is acceptable to you, what places, if any, there are for young people to congregate; whether or not a car is required to get there; and other factors.

2. **When is it okay for your teen to go out solo with another person?** This one is tougher; when is it okay for your adolescent to date another person in a one-to-one relationship? One aspect of your decision is to consider the age of the person that your child wishes to date, or the upper limit that you would find acceptable. For example, you may not want your child to date another person who is more than two or three years older than the child. In addition, keep in mind that in many cases of teenage pregnancies, the male partner was often in his twenties or older.

The maturity of your teen is another issue. Is a 16-year-old boy really ready to date a 19-year-old female college student? Maybe not, although he may be certain he is.

3. **What curfew is reasonable?** Many parents set a curfew for when the teenager must be in the house, and often that curfew is earlier on "school nights" than it is on holidays or weekends. What curfew is best for your child should be discussed with him or her, keeping in mind that the adolescent would prefer to have no curfew at all!

Sexual behavior

Your children probably learned in elementary school how babies are conceived, and they know the technical terms as well as the obscene ones. What they may not know is what you believe is okay or not okay. So tell your child. Does this mean that you must tell your child about your own current or former sexual behavior? Some moms with ADD may have had a rather exciting past.

Most children are repelled by the idea of their parents having ever had sex—except to conceive them. Retain your privacy. Whether you tell your children about previous sexual behavior is up to you, but there is no obligation to do so.

If you disapprove of intercourse for teens, then say so. Do be explicit about what creates pregnancy or prevents it. Knowing something doesn't mean a child will feel compelled to act it out. Your children may not have been listening during the lecture on birth control—especially if they have ADD! It is likely that they will listen to you, if only out of shock and curiosity about what you will say.

Schoolwork

Everyone wants their children to get good grades, but the fact is that school is easy for some children and hard for others (read the next chapter, "School Daze").

If your child does his or her homework and maintains at least average grades, that may be the best she can do, especially if she has ADD. You may wish to request that accommodations be made to her ADD, but don't assume her grades will skyrocket as a result.

Parenting an adolescent is not a job for the faint-hearted. The mom with ADD may be prone to remember how she was as a teenager and allow her teen too much freedom, or she may tighten the reins a little too much. In this chapter, I covered common adolescent behaviors and discussed the importance of considering boundaries and expectations—yours and theirs.

10

School Daze: Your Child Goes to School

Many say that the one area where they run into the most problems is school. Whether or not your child has ADD, often you find that you reach accommodations with each other and have your own routines and ways of coping. But eventually, when your child is five or six, it's time for your baby to go off to school.

In this chapter, you'll find some solutions to common "school daze" problems such as these:

- Helping your child adjust
- Organizing school paperwork for you and your child
- Dealing with typical problems that arise in school
- Attending parent-teacher conferences
- Finishing homework and science projects and getting them in on time

This chapter also includes information about alternatives to public schools (charter schools and home schooling). It concludes with a discussion of school requirements for children with ADD, and a look at what to do if the school refuses to cooperate in evaluating your child for learning disabilities.

▶ HELPING YOUR CHILD ADJUST

School can be difficult whether your child is six or sixteen, for different reasons. You'll find that whether it's learning to spell *cat* or *logarithm*, the challenges and frustrations can be very similar. Of course, how you handle these challenges should be adapted to the child's developmental level. A five-year-old may just need a hug, but a teenager may cringe or even leap back in horror if offered the same. They don't want to be treated like a "baby" by you.

Starting Out: Excited Children and Crying Moms

The first time your "baby" goes to kindergarten is a very exciting time—and also a very emotional time for most mothers and even some fathers. Kindergarten teachers are used to seeing adult women with tears running down their faces, reluctant to turn over their little girl or boy to a stranger. Even if the child has been attending a childcare center for years, it's still different—maybe because entering school seems so official as well as being a rite of passage for a child.

Sometimes children are fearful of school too, and it doesn't help much if Mom is as clingy as the child. In most cases, either the first day or in a few days, children rapidly adjust to kindergarten.

Demands School Places on Children: Homework Hassles and Other Issues

If you feel like you're being eaten alive by your kid's homework, there's something wrong and that's a real barometer. It means that you're off balance, you have taken on too much of the problem.
—Kate Kelly, a prominent ADD coach and author of several important books on ADD

I agree with Kelly and think that for many of us, homework is a tricky issue. If your child has ADD too, you may be in for a challenging time. Work to have someone else get involved with this part of your child's life. Either ask your spouse to work with the child or hire a high school student to help, especially if your child is as disorganized as you are.

If your child has significant difficulty with school and you can't provide the help he needs, consider a tutor. There is no reason why you should expect yourself to somehow "know" how to teach tasks like reading or doing algebraic equations.

Everything In Its Place: But What Place Is That?

When I forget to send in things like gift-wrap orders, homework papers, etc., teachers have always always been condescending. As much as I understand and accept my ADD myself, I've yet to overcome feeling incredibly small in the eyes of the teachers who just don't understand that adults/moms can also have ADD.
—Lynn, 37, mother of one daughter

When your child goes to school, be prepared for reams of paper, much of it looking absolutely useless, and arriving home from school, starting with Day One. Because many ADD moms are hoarders, they won't throw away these sheets, although they may have major trouble finding papers the teachers want. How do moms know what is to be saved? Or turned back in to the teacher? You ask the teacher.

If your child has ADD, you have probably encountered this phenomenon: The probability that your child will lose a school paper is directly related to its importance; that is, the more important it is, the more likely it is to be lost. This is complicated by the fact that even if he doesn't lose the paper, you might, because of *your* ADD!

If this is a chronic problem and nothing you've tried works, ask the teacher if she can mail really important forms to you, or see if she can fax them—and give her your fax number. You may encounter a little resistance. However, it can be an annoying problem for the teacher to keep track of papers that are not returned, and you could ask the teacher if that's true for her. One secret of obtaining cooperation from teachers (or anyone else) is finding an advantage to them as well as to you.

VERY SIMPLE HOMEWORK CHECKLIST

Use this checklist and/or adapt it for your needs. When you make your child's checklist, be sure the items are in BIG LETTERS, no matter how old your child is. Then hang it, tape it, or post it in a place your child can't miss it—even if it's the bathroom.

- Did you write your name on it?
- Did you write today's date on it?
- Did you write the subject on it?
- Does the teacher want his or her name on it?
- Did you put it in your backpack, by the front door, or somewhere easy to remember?
- Are you sure you did the right assignment?

▶ IF PROBLEMS ARISE

Even though my daughter was diagnosed with ADD at age 9, most teachers still thought more effort was the key. Also, because so many articles have been written about the over-diagnosis of ADD, they jump to that conclusion when you have a very bright child who isn't bouncing off walls.
—Bonnie, 41, mother of two teenagers

Believe it or not, non-ADD mothers can struggle with problems at school too—although your struggles may seem worse because your ADD complicates your responses. Here are a few possible problems that you may find yourself facing.

1. **The neat-aholic teacher.** Most teachers are normal, nice people; but once in awhile, you'll run across Ms. Rigidity, who wants everything done just so. And it's "my way or the highway" as far as she is concerned—the only one right way to do things is whatever way she dictates. Ms. Rigidity can be quite a problem for the mom with ADD!

If you know about this teacher in advance, ask for a different teacher. If you can't change teachers, try to negotiate with Ms. Rigidity so that you can work together.

2. **The accusatory teacher.** More than one of the mothers I interviewed said they faced a situation in which, during a parent-teacher conference, the teacher suddenly said, "Mrs. Jones, would you *please* sit still? Now I know where your son gets it from!" The mothers were so horrified and upset by this outburst that they were nearly paralyzed, and the meeting went precipitously downhill from there.

What could a person say in such an instance? Well, first of all, if the teacher used a talking-down tone of voice, it would be good to remind her that you are an adult, after all.

If you are feeling confident about your own ADD, you might say something like this: "That's interesting that you mentioned my moving about, because I do have a bit of ADD myself and so I can understand why my son has it too. In fact, many parents have ADD themselves. Sometimes it's easier for people like us to be able to move about or stand because it can be hard for us to sit still."

Whatever your response, try to make it an adult-to-adult answer. Just because a teacher talked down to you does not mean that you must respond as a child. Realize that you're a grown-up, and the teacher needs to respect you as an adult.

Reasonable and Unreasonable Demands Teachers and Schools Can Make

Sometimes the school system itself may make unreasonable demands; for example, the starting time for school in one city in Florida was made later only after several children were run over and killed on crowded dark streets where the bus picked them up.

You don't have to wait for the school to realize it has a serious problem. If you as a parent can see that it's nuts to expect five-year-old Johnny to walk two miles to school, then say so. Talk to elected officials. Write letters to the editor. You are your child's best advocate—or should be! The "squeaky wheel" really does get the grease, especially when you have a legitimate complaint.

▶ PARENT-TEACHER CONFERENCES

Some parents dread parent-teacher conferences more than they do addressing coworkers in a formal presentation. Both are hard. But in the case of the parent-teacher conference, sometimes you will hear some critical or negative information about your child, and you may "hear" an underlying criticism of your own parenting. That can be tough to take.

There are basically two possible scenarios, the benevolent conference and the problem conference. For each type of conference, you should be as prepared and ready to listen and communicate as possible:

1. **Write down your primary concerns.** You don't want to forget them—and yes, you can forget them during the actual meeting. The teacher may attempt to dominate you, or you may become distracted. Make the list. And bring it with you.

2. **Think about what you should wear to the meeting.** Appearances do count. If you normally wear jeans and a shirt (as I do), dress up for the parent-teacher meeting. No, you don't have to wear a ball gown and a tiara. But wear clothing suitable to a meeting between professionals: a dress, a suit, or a pantsuit.

3. **Remind yourself that this meeting is not about *you*.** (Although you want to make a good impression.) The main issue is your child. You are your child's primary advocate. Maybe you don't like schools and you don't like meetings. But you need to do what is best for your child.

4. **Go in with an open mind.** Your child may have painted his teacher(s) as truly awful and overbearing. Maybe they are. But maybe that is his perception. However, also keep in mind that teachers act differently with parents than they do with children.

Read the section on effective listening in "Juggling Family and Work: The Family (Chapter Four), which provides specific hints that apply to a teacher conference or a meeting with anyone you need to interact with and communicate important information.

ARE TEACHERS UNDERSTANDING OF MOMS WITH ADD?

Here's what some ADD moms say:

- They expect me to teach skills to my son that I haven't mastered yet myself. I am very disorganized and it is very difficult to teach by example what you cannot do.

- The school refused to remind my daughter to get her Ritalin. Their answer was for me to come to school every day at noon and give her the Ritalin.

- Maybe some are, but my recent experiences with my son's teacher have not been very kind or understanding.

- I am not sure, because I haven't told my children's teachers that I have ADD. I'm afraid they wouldn't take me seriously when I try to get something for my son with ADD.

- There's always pressure to go to PTA meetings, make cookies, participate in fundraisers, help my child with homework, keep her organized—it's very hard because I can barely keep my own head above water.

- Teachers make comments like "the apple doesn't fall far from the tree," but don't understand why that makes it so difficult—it's biological, not willful.

- I am a teacher and often hear other teachers complain about moms who can't seem to pull it together. Of course, maybe the mothers have not been diagnosed with ADD, but they seem to struggle with some of the same difficulties as their children.

- When I forget to send in things like gift-wrap orders, homework papers, etc., the teachers have *always* been condescending.

- Teachers always discuss ADD as a child's problem or a parenting problem. I don't think they know this problem continues into adulthood.

- I don't think they have enough experience with kids with ADD, let alone with their mothers.

▶ HOMEWORK HEADACHES AND SCIENCE PROJECT NIGHTMARES

If you have ADD and your child has ADD too, homework hassles can get you down. Long-term projects, such as science fair projects or tasks that must be done over weeks or months, can feel like they will be your undoing. There are some ways to mitigate the madness, however.

SCHOOL MODIFICATIONS FOR CHILDREN WITH ADD

If your child has ADD, it may be extremely helpful if basic modifications are made to the classroom, or if tools such as tape recorders are allowed in class. According to a memorandum issued by the U.S. Department of Education in 1991, the following are possible modifications for children who have ADD:

"Providing a structured learning environment; repeating and simplifying instructions about in-class and homework assignments; supplementing verbal instructions with visual instructions; using behavioral management techniques; adjusting class schedules; modifying test delivery; using tape recorders, computer-aided instruction, and other audiovisual equipment; selecting modified textbooks or workbooks; and tailoring homework assignments. Other provisions range from consultation to special recourse and may include reducing class size; use of one-on-one tutorials, classroom aides and note takers; involvement of a 'services coordinator' to oversee implementation of special programs and services, and possible modification of nonacademic items such as lunchroom, recess, and physical education."

Surviving Science Projects and Homework Headaches

When you have ADD, it's hard to plan ahead for three months from now, although that may be the timeframe over which a science project is due.

Of course, you may not find out about the project until two days before it's due. Be sure to ask your children about schoolwork *every day,* so you can discover this information in advance. A lot of times you'll receive noncommittal answers; but keep asking, and eventually you will find out what you need to know.

Also, if the teacher or the school sends home a newsletter, be sure to read it right away, when the child pulls it out from her backpack. Don't leave it on the kitchen counter, planning to "read it later." Ha! By then it will be lost or spilled on.

Knowing that many children can't plan as far ahead as three months, some schools require that parts of the project are due on specific dates. For example, first the hypothesis, then the description of the project, and so forth until the actual final project must be brought in.

Here's my advice on science projects, especially for the mom with ADD:

- **Keep the idea simple.** Negotiate with the child a project that you both can live with.

- **Keep the materials simple.** You should not have to spend lots of money on a science project. Some parents do but I think they are making a mistake.

- **Make sure it's something that a visual display can be made for, and that it's not too disgusting.** One year we measured mold and brought in mold samples. Mega yuck!

- **Don't do all the work for your child.** For the overeager parent, including the mom with ADD, it may seem much easier to do it yourself. Resist this impulse. Make sure she or he learns something from this project and can understand it and explain it.

- **Ask for help.** Check with your friends, relatives, or neighbors without kids—they may view the science project as fun—and your child will enjoy the extra attention. You may also be able to trade something with them: They help your child with the project, and you house-sit for them when they go away for the weekend.

Homework Ideas

Check to see that your child has the materials she needs to do homework. Also, if your child has ADD, it's best to have her do her homework in a place where she can be monitored, such as the kitchen table. If she's in her room, you may think she's working hard at her desk, while she's really playing instead.

Is your child overloaded with homework? Yes, if your child is spending three or more hours on homework every night—unless she's in college. Maybe the work is too hard for your child, and she should not be in advanced or gifted classes. Maybe the teachers are too heavy-handed with homework. Many children as young as 10 can have three or more teachers. If these teachers don't talk to each other, they may not realize how much they are loading down children.

You may need to help your child with homework, but don't do everything for your child. I won't write my children's essays for them. I'll offer suggestions and listen to their ideas and maybe even type an essay. But I want them to learn how to compose.

The same is true for math, social studies, and other subjects. If you do all the homework for the child, he won't learn—and he will do poorly on tests and quizzes. Have the child offer to teach *you* the math problem. If you don't understand it, ask questions. Many of us actually learn information better by teaching it to others.

ADD expert and psychologist Kathleen Nadeau says that in some schools, homework assignments are posted on the school website, and she favors this. As a result, if your child forgets or loses his homework assignment, he can look it up and know what is to be done—rather than frantically trying to reconstruct it from memory.

The next section covers a rapidly growing new educational opportunity for children nationwide: the charter school.

▶ WHEN THE SYSTEM IS NOT THE SOLUTION: CHARTER SCHOOLS MAY WORK

It's important to advocate for your child as much as possible. This may mean working hard with your child's teachers and making sure needed accommodations are made to homework, curriculum, and so forth. But one problem is that no matter how effective you are at advocating, there will still be some teachers and administrators in the "regular" school who don't understand ADD and who don't even believe that it's a real problem—for children or adults.

If you're exhausted from fighting an uphill battle with the school and are wondering if the system is really the solution, maybe it isn't. Maybe a charter school would be a good choice for your child who has ADD or a learning disability. These are schools within the public school system, but created by a person or group of people who have an often impassioned interest in a particular group of children. They work very hard to obtain a "charter," so that they can open and run a school for the children they would like to help.

Not all charter schools are specifically oriented to children with ADD, but many are. And since they were created to work with children with ADD or other problems—or sometimes several different problems—they believe and they know that ADD is real. They are also more willing to work with families. For example, Lana, 43, told me that the charter school administrators at the school her daughter attends said they knew that kids with ADD frequently lose school papers and important notes for parents. They had a policy of calling parents to make sure important documents were received. Non-charter schools can't do this, because they have too many students. Nor would they see any reason why they should do this. And in most cases, they would be right. But we are talking about your child with ADD, not anyone else's child.

What Are Charter Schools?

Charter schools are operated by private organizations or individuals and receive public school funds. They are nonsectarian (nonreligious) schools and must comply with state and federal civil rights, health, and safety laws and regulations. Charter schools vary in their mission. There are schools for gifted students, vocational students, and for children with learning disabilities or ADD. Some schools specialize in helping children who have serious emotional problems.

Many people have little or no knowledge of charter schools, but despite this, the charter school concept is one of the hottest educational trends in the United States today.

In 1999, President Clinton announced more than $95 million in three-year federal grants to nineteen states, the District of Columbia, and Puerto Rico. These grants were awarded to help meet the growing demand for public charter schools and stemmed from the Charter Schools Expansion Act of 1998, enacted by Congress. The president's goal was to increase the number of charter schools from about 1,200 in 1998 to 3,000 by 2002. As of March 2000, there were about 1,700 charter schools attended by about 250,000 children in 27 states and the District of Columbia.

Where Are Charter Schools?

The first charter school legislation was passed in Minnesota in 1991, followed by legislation in California in 1992. As of 1999, thirty-six states have passed charter school laws, with the most recent entrants (1999) as of this writing being Oklahoma and Oregon. Not all of the states that have passed laws actually have schools in place as of early 2000 (see the state-by-state chart at the end of this section.)

How old are the children who attend charter schools? Charter schools may accommodate children from kindergarten through grade twelve, depending on state laws and requirements. (See Appendix G in this book for state contacts to learn more about charter schools.)

State-by-State Chart on Charter Schools as of January 2000

State	Charter School Law Passed? If so, when?	Number of Charter Schools
Alabama	No	
Alaska	Yes, 1995	18 schools
Arkansas	Yes, 1995	None so far
California	Yes, 1992	234 schools
Colorado	Yes, 1993	69 schools
Connecticut	Yes, 1996	17 schools
District of Columbia	Yes, 1996	29 schools
Delaware	Yes, 1995	5 schools

State	Charter School Law Passed? If so, when?	Number of Charter Schools
Florida	Yes, 1996	112 schools
Georgia	Yes, 1993	32 schools
Hawaii	Yes, 1994	2 schools
Idaho	Yes, 1998	8 schools
Illinois	Yes, 1996	17 schools
Indiana	No	
Iowa	No	
Kansas	Yes, 1994	15 schools
Kentucky	No	
Louisiana	Yes, 1995	24 schools
Maine	No	
Maryland	No	
Massachusetts	Yes, 1993	34 schools
Michigan	Yes, 1993	175*
Minnesota	Yes, 1991	55 schools
Missouri	Yes, 1998	15 schools
Mississippi	Yes, 1997	1 school
Montana	No	
New Hampshire	Yes, 1995	None so far
New Jersey	Yes, 1996	50 schools
New Mexico	Yes, 1993	5 schools
New York	Yes, 1998	5 schools
Nevada	Yes, 1997	2 schools
North Carolina	Yes, 1996	86 schools
North Dakota	No	
Ohio	Yes, 1997	48 schools
Oklahoma	Yes, 1999	None yet
Oregon	Yes, 1999	16 schools
Pennsylvania	Yes, 1997	49 schools
Rhode Island	Yes, 1995	2 schools
South Carolina	Yes, 1996	10 schools
South Dakota	No	
Texas	Yes, 1995	150 schools
Utah	Yes, 1998	8 schools

State	Charter School Law Passed? If so, when?	Number of Charter Schools
Vermont	No	
Virginia	Yes, 1998	None yet
Washington	No	
West Virginia	No	
Wisconsin	Yes, 1993	35 schools
Wyoming	Yes, 1995	None yet
Puerto Rico	Yes, (don't have date approved)	62 schools

* Michigan calls its charter schools *public school academies.*

Pros and Cons of Charter Schools

Skeptics and those who believe that only traditional schools are acceptable for children have several fears. Primary among them is the fear that charter schools will take funds away from traditional public schools; however, supporters say that charter schools accommodate children that the traditional schools have failed. Another fear has been that charter schools would take only the very best students and leave behind students with disabilities. In fact, most charter schools do include children with disabilities. Some schools specialize in helping children with learning disabilities, attention deficit disorder, and other problems. Some states require that charter schools concentrate on children with disabilities. In most charter schools, classes are much smaller than in traditional schools.

Another concern was that White children would dominate charter schools, and minorities would be left behind. In contrast to fears that charter schools would leave minority students behind, studies of charter schools by the U.S. Department of Education have found that such schools are racially balanced, and many have a heavy concentration of children with disabilities or other special needs. In fact, in some states, charter schools must concentrate on such children or enroll a substantial number of them.

One "con" that has presented a problem in some states is that new charter schools may struggle financially. The founders need to comply with state and federal regulations, and they are often on a limited budget. They do receive state funds, but often they have a much lower teacher-student ratio than the public school, which means more teachers. Sometimes teachers, uncertain if the school will continue to operate next year or the year after, may be reluctant to work for a charter school. In contrast, traditional public schools are assumed to continue on indefinitely as long as the child population needs the schools.

There are a variety of other pros and cons, and the key points are summarized in the following chart.

	Traditional Public School	Charter School
Funding	State and federal funds.	State, federal, and private funds.
Leaders/Founders	Principal of school.	Founders/leaders may or may not be educational experts and may have a learning curve to contend with.
Type of Students	All types: gifted, average, and children needing special services.	Varies, although most concentrate on a particular student population and many schools accommodate children with attention deficit disorder, learning disabilities, and other needs.
Track Record	Often have been around for years. Some parents are satisfied, while others are very dissatisfied.	A new entrant, launched in the 1990s and still trying to prove itself.
Class Sizes	Standard large classes: Median school sizes are 500 students.	Usually are small classes: Median number of students in school is 150 students.
Transportation	Buses usually provided.	Transportation sometimes not available.
Curriculum	Traditional curriculum, in general.	May be traditional, although many use innovative techniques.

Did Charter Schools Spring Up from Nowhere?

Some charter schools were traditional schools that were converted to a charter school to accommodate a specific population of students. Other charter schools were created in response to federal and state legislation and a perceived need of students for such schools.

In general, charter schools are given goals to meet, and they are monitored by state agencies. However, the level of autonomy the schools enjoy seems to vary greatly from state to state and possibly within the states as well.

Why Are Few Parents Aware of Charter Schools?

Many parents have no idea that charter schools may be operating in their own home state and even in their own city. I think one reason is that they seem to receive little media attention.

I learned that there were several charter schools in my community that specifically concentrated on elementary and middle-school children with attention deficit disorder and/or learning disabilities. In addition, other charter schools provided vocational training for high school students. Charter schools became so popular that the school board in my area appointed a full-time person to administer charter schools. I also learned that there were waiting lists to get into some of the charter schools, because parents were so eager for their children to enter.

Another key advantage of charter schools is that parents need not pay additional funds for their children to attend, because the schools already receive public school funds. In addition, the charter schools may offer programs or services that even private schools may not provide.

A down side of charter schools is that parents may be expected to volunteer time, because schools may operate on a shoestring. In addition, because school buses may not available, parents must find transportation to and from the school for their children. These constraints have not discouraged charter school supporters.

One thing you generally cannot do is find an entry for "charter schools" in the Yellow Pages of your telephone book, because they are usually included under the category of all public schools. Thus, if you don't know the specific name of a charter school, you would not know how to locate and identify it.

To Learn More

If you'd like more information about whether there are charter schools in your state, county, or city, it's best to contact the organization that administers schools in your area. The principal of the local elementary school may know about charter schools in the area—and may also perceive them as competition. You can also contact the education department in your state.

The U.S. Education Department has information on charter schools, including reports on the schools, on the Internet. The General Accounting Office has also analyzed nationwide charter schools, and this information also can be accessed online. You could also contact the governor's office in your state to request information on charter schools.

▶ HOME SCHOOLING

This is a very short section, because I could find nothing on home schooling in relation to moms with ADD. In fact, it seems to me that home schooling would be very difficult for a mother who has ADD herself. At one point my son asked me to home school him, and I nearly burst into laughter. I know teaching a child takes a certain regimen and structure, and I also knew it was beyond my capabilities. I told him that it was really not a good idea, because I didn't know how to teach children and didn't think I could learn it, especially "on the job."

It is possible that some might be able to handle home schooling. One mother did tell me that she was home-schooling her children. I suspect, however, that for most of us, it's not a very good idea.

▶ IF YOUR CHILD HAS ADD: SCHOOL REQUIREMENTS

Many people have said to me, aren't there federal laws that the schools have to comply with? Answer: Yes, of course there are. That does not mean that they will necessarily comply with these laws. They may not wish to expend the extra effort. Or they may not be aware of federal laws, although ignorance of the law is no excuse. As a result, sometimes moms have to advocate for their children, and that can mean sticking your neck out. That can be hard! But it is worth it.

Key Federal Requirements

The main federal law you need to know about in relation to your child and school is the Individuals with Disabilities Education Act (IDEA), although Section 504 and the Americans with Disabilities Act of 1990 may also be relevant to your child.

A Good IDEA

IDEA's predecessor, the Education for All Handicapped Children Act, has been around since 1975; however, children with attention deficit disorder were not specifically mentioned and were only alluded to in a 1991 policy memorandum issued by the Department of Education. The good news is that the bill that was reauthorized by Congress and signed into law by President Clinton does specifically include children with ADD. The regulations that were released in March of 1999 listed ADD as an "other health impairment." The language reads as follows:

> Other health impairment means having limited strength, vitality or alertness, including a heightened alertness to environmental stimuli, that results in limited alertness with respect to the educational environment, that:
>> (i) is due to chronic or acute health problems such as asthma, attention deficit disorder or attention deficit hyperactivity disorder, diabetes, epilepsy, a heart condition, hemophilia, lead poising, leukemia, nephritis, rheumatic fever, and sickle cell anemia; and
>> (ii) adversely affects a child's educational performance.

If your child qualifies for IDEA, then the guidance department of the school will work with you and the child's teachers to prepare an Individual Education Plan (IEP). The plan will be discussed at a meeting with you, and a formal written plan will be worked out.

Your child may not need special services, and yet you may feel that he needs some accommodations to the problems that can be caused by ADD. In that, case, you may find that Section 504 of the Rehabilitation Act of 1973 would be more applicable.

Section 504

Section 504 is another federal provision that may apply to your child. This is actually a civil-rights law and is Section 504 of the Rehabilitation Act of 1973. It requires schools to "make a free and appropriate public education" available to students with disabilities when educational performance is affected—and ADD is considered a disability. The emphasis is on regular class attendance with some modifications, such as sitting close to the teacher, tape-recording classes, and receiving other accommodations worked out in advance.

Whether it would be better to go for IDEA or Section 504 is beyond the scope of this book; however, they are two separate and distinct laws. If, for example, your child doesn't seem to "fit" within the parameters of IDEA, he or she may fit those of Section 504 instead. You may need only a physician's diagnosis for Section 504, whereas IDEA may require more formal testing; however, state laws and policies vary.

The Americans with Disabilities Act of 1990

I've also talked about the Americans with Disabilities Act in "Juggling Family and Work: The Workplace (Chapter Five) on making it work at work. But the fact is that the federal law that may apply to your child with ADD is the Americans with Disabilities Act of 1990. This law prohibits discrimination against people, including students, with disabilities; and it is applicable to all public schools. Most experts believe it is virtually interchangeable with Section 504 in its impact on children in school.

According to author Robert R. Erk, an associate professor of counselor education in his 1999 article for *Professional School Counseling*:

Children and adolescents with ADHD are presently covered by the following three federal acts or statutes: (a) the Individuals with Disabilities Education Act, Part B (IDEA); (b) Section 504 of the Rehabilitation Act of 1973; and (c) the Americans with Disabilities Act of 1990 (ADA). School personnel should be aware that the U.S. Department of Education has the legal authority to interpret and enforce IDEA, and the department's Office of Civil Rights interprets and enforces the education related provisions of Section 504 and ADA.

Types of Educational Accommodations

Many kinds of educational accommodations are possible. Here are some examples of accommodations to ADD:

- Assigning less homework
- Allowing child to type his or her homework on the computer
- Giving the child more time to take tests
- Providing extra warnings about assignments

Will My Child Be Stigmatized If We Ask for Assistance?

Many parents worry that their child may be seen as "stupid" or mentally ill if they request extra help. This probably dates back to decades ago, when the only children in special education were children who were developmentally delayed. But today, many more children have been designated as having a need for extra help. In fact, even "gifted" children are designated as children with special needs because of their high intelligence.

If you are thinking about asking the school if your child qualifies for one of the federal programs, ask yourself:

1. Is my child struggling in school? If the child is receiving A's and B's, he may not need any extra help. If, however, he is doing below-average or failing work, then you may be throwing him a lifeline by getting him into the IDEA or 504 program.

2. Is the teacher likely to notice my child's disability? The teacher will probably realize if your child is not doing well; however, if the child is not hyperactive and is instead primarily inattentive, this problem is often unrecognized, even by good teachers.

3. How is your child's self-esteem? Feeling upset about school performance and "dumb" can adversely affect your child, even for the long term. Many adults with ADD report how miserable they were with teachers who berated them and made no allowances for them at all. Certainly if your child's self-esteem could be raised by some accommodations, you should consider that option.

4. Are you embarrassed because you don't want your child to be identified as a child who needs help? This is common, but the basic answer is: Get over it.

Sample Letter to Guidance Counselor

The following letter and the form that I created should be adapted by you to fit your own child's situation, and only if you feel that going in and talking to the guidance counselor may not work. For example, you may wish to have all teachers sign the form, or you may have other needs that I have not addressed here. As you consider how to modify the form so that it will be best for your child, remember this: Let "Keep It Simple, Silly" (KISS) be your guide.

October 10, 2000

Dear Counselor:

I am the mother of [name of child] and I am very concerned with his school performance. I know that I need to discuss this issue with you on the phone or in person, but I wanted to express my concerns in writing first.

The problem that [name of child] faces is that he is doing poorly in several subjects because he either forgets to do his homework, or he does the work and does not hand it in. These are classic features of a child with attention deficit disorder and my son has been diagnosed with this disorder. He is primarily forgetful and inattentive. [Name of child] has an educational plan in his school record but has not wanted any special treatment and has been struggling to remember to do his work. Clearly, he needs some accommodation. Fortunately, attention deficit disorder continues to be a disability specifically cited by the federal government as one that may necessitate accommodations and that is cited in the regulations written in May of 1999. It's also my understanding that the bill President Clinton signed expanded this accommodation requirement.

I think that [name of child]'s teachers are doing a great job and hope they will understand the need for this accommodation to my son's disability. In my opinion, my requested action could mean the difference between [name of child]'s passing or failing.

I am hoping that you would consider requesting that my child's teachers in the following subjects (list them) use the simple form I'm enclosing with this letter. If they will let me know on a daily basis, through this form, whether my child is doing work or not, and if not, what should be done to make it up, I would appreciate it.

I would like to discuss this problem with you at your earliest convenience.

Thank you.

Sincerely,

[Your Name]

Daily Schoolwork Form for [Name of Child]

Name of Teacher: _____   Date:_____

1. As far as you know, did [name of child] complete the
work that you expected to be done in class today?   Yes   No

2. If [name of child] did not do classwork today, what can
(he/she) do to make up what was not done?

_____

_____

3. Did [name of child] turn in homework that was due today?   Yes   No

4. If [name of child] did not turn in (his/her) homework, what work was due that he should make up?

_____

_____

5. Any comments or suggestions?

_____

_____

_____

▶ **IF THE SCHOOL ABSOLUTELY REFUSES TO COOPERATE: WHAT ONE PARENT TRIED THAT WORKED**

Sometimes it happens. Even though you have federal and state law on your side, and even though your child has been diagnosed with ADD and is clearly struggling and needing help, the school may refuse to provide an evaluation of your child. Or, more frequently, they may delay, delay, delay.

"I waited six months for my daughter to be tested and every day, her self-esteem seemed to sink a little lower," said Eve, 32, mother of Tiffany, an eight-year-old girl. Finally, Eve decided that the school was probably never going to test Tiffany, and she might even fail the second grade. Eve had talked to the school principal and received vague promises of later, urging to be "patient," and so forth.

She finally decided she had had it when Tiffany came home one day and said everyone thought she was stupid because she couldn't read as well as the others. The child said she didn't know why, but sometimes she got so interested in looking out the window that she forgot what she was supposed to be working on. Eve told Tiffany she most definitely was _not_ stupid.

The next day, Eve did some investigating. She found out that Tiffany was entitled to be evaluated for learning disabilities, and she also learned that ADD was considered to be a category of disability for children with ADD who were struggling and met other criteria.

Eve typed up a letter to the superintendent of schools, and stated that she felt Tiffany was being discriminated against because of her disability. Eve referred to the federal legislation, IDEA, and the Americans with Disabilities Act.

She enclosed a copy of a letter from Tiffany's doctor, stating that the child definitely had ADD and her inattentiveness did require her to have accommodations.

Eve worried briefly that she or her child might "get in trouble," but decided that things were so bad that she had to do something. She mailed the letter, sending it certified return receipt so that nobody could claim that it never arrived. Two days later, Eve received a call. Her daughter's testing would be next week. In addition, a meeting to make a plan for needed accommodations for Tiffany would be held the following week. Her teacher and the guidance counselor would attend.

The testing revealed some learning difficulties, although not severe ones. However, Tiffany's ADD was clearly holding her back, and a meeting was scheduled to create the "Individualized Education Plan" for Tiffany.

Eve was a little nervous the day of the meeting. She and Tiffany both attended. Her nervousness increased when she saw the principal come into the room, obviously planning on sitting in on this meeting. Eve was a little intimidated.

But things went well. All Eve really wanted was feedback, preferably daily feedback from the teacher that Tiffany was doing her work. She also wanted to receive, in writing, information on any homework that was assigned. She wanted to know if Tiffany was experiencing any serious problems, and she wanted to know in a timely manner—the week, if not the day, problems happened, rather than weeks later when she couldn't do anything about it.

Eve got exactly what she wanted, and everyone seemed satisfied. No one seemed angry, although Eve later wondered *why* she had to go to such extremes to receive simple accommodations.

In this chapter, I discussed how many moms with ADD struggled in school because they were inattentive or bored. When their children complain about school, moms with ADD may remember their own problems and sometimes they rush in and help too much. The good news is there are workable strategies. In addition, if your child has ADD, the law is on her side.

The charter school, covered in this chapter, is a new opportunity for many students with ADD throughout the nation. These schools provide specialized help for children with learning disabilities, ADD and other problems. And since they receive state and federal funds, charter schools don't charge tuition.

PART THREE

Special Struggles

The next section covers the major struggle many moms with ADD face in dealing with the emotions that our ADD can generate. Sometimes these emotions are very dark. How do you cope with sheer rage? Or hopelessness and helplessness?

In addition, sometimes it is particular times that try mother's hearts and souls, although these times vary from person to person. For one person, it may be Christmas, which should be perfect—like when she was 10 years old. For another person, it could be a trip in the car with the kids.

11

Coping with Difficult or Painful Emotions that May Accompany ADD

**I hate the rage and frustration I sometimes feel
when my daughters act up. It mostly happens
at night when the day has taken its toll on me
and my mind is just plain tired out.**
—Jeanine, 27, mother of one

Sometimes it's the painful emotions or the stress that can accompany ADD that bother moms more than anything else. Moms feel one way but they think that they "should" feel another way. So they become angry with themselves and get stuck in a negative loop of mentally beating up on themselves. They may also become depressed and find themselves drawing inward.

They "know" no one else is like them, and they may also be convinced that all other Moms know special secrets that help them control their behavior, secrets that are somehow unknowable or at least unknown by the mom with ADD.

Previous chapters have covered dealing with your children's problematic behavior. But what if the person with the overflowing cauldron of emotions is you? This chapter looks at these difficult and very common emotions and offers suggestions on how to cope with feelings and deal with the difficult emotions common to many moms with ADD, including:

- Corraling your temper over a child's misbehavior
- Limiting your own feelings of self-blame and guilt
- Coping with frustration and feeling incompetent
- Keeping your stress levels down
- Mastering feeling overwhelmed
- Challenging feelings that ADD automatically makes you a bad mother
- Learning what real bad mothers are like

- Considering whether an emotional issue may be impeding your parenting

Anger or rage, followed later by major feelings of guilt, can occur when the mom with ADD becomes overwhelmed by life's problems. Combine the normal frustration of a bad day with one or more tired, whining children and you have serious potential for a major meltdown. Yet you need to learn how to get a handle on common emotions.

"OUTWARDLY CALM"

"I have a sign on my computer that says, 'Outwardly Calm,' and it often really does help me when I glance at it," says Tammy, 42, mother of two. She says if she acts calm, it helps her to feel calm.

A subsidiary problem of anger and overreacting is that the ADD Mom often may feel guilty and contrite and rescind whatever punishment she had assigned for a child's behavioral infraction. The trouble is, the kids usually know this is a pattern for Mom.

Rage: When You Feel Yourself "Losing It"

Anger is a very strong emotion, but "losing it" is stronger—we're talking rage here, sheer and blind. We may not like these feelings one iota but nearly everyone at some point in time has found herself in the middle of a blinding rage, somewhat like a toddler's temper tantrum. Except we are bigger and can cause a lot more damage than our two-year-old ever could.

It's not only children who need to be sent to their rooms for exploding emotions or misbehavior. Sometimes Mom finds herself spilling over with emotion and the anger and yelling come pouring out.

When you feel yourself losing it, send yourself to your room for a five-minute time-out. In just five minutes, you can often regain your calmness and begin again. If the children are old enough to understand, tell them you're taking a time-out. If they're infants or toddlers, you may need to put them in a crib or other safe place until you pull yourself together.

Coping with Anger: Your Own Personal Emotional Anchor

Sometimes it can help considerably if you create an emotional anchor for yourself, during those times when you feel fine. What the heck is an emotional anchor? To me, it's a way to regain emotional control when you start to feel overly angry, overly upset, and overly frustrated. For many people, their emotional anchor can be an image.

Doreen, 32, says she has a special place in her mind that she returns to when she needs to calm herself. "If I am overtired or overly distraught, I think about a riverbank I knew as a child. It was a place where I always felt safe and calm. I imagine the scene of the water rushing over the flattened-down rocks. I imagine hearing the bubbly kind of sound the water made as it rushed along. I imagine how cold and pure the water felt."

This may not work for you. Try imaging another scene, or even imaging yourself petting your cat or doing some other activity. The key is that it should be an activity that is calming, not exciting.

Don't pound on pillows when you're really mad. Psychiatrists say that this just promotes the idea that hitting something will make you feel better. Instead, try running up and down the stairs or around the house a few times.

▶ SELF-BLAME AND GUILT

**My house is a mess and I never invite people
over because of it. I feel guilty because I don't
have the June Cleaver image.**
—Alicia, 36, mother of a five-year-old son

Guilt and self-blame can become very prominent emotions in the lives of mothers who have ADD.

"I feel guilty and inadequate sometimes when I do things I do *not* believe in, such as yelling at my child, and I do not do things that I value greatly, such as sticking to a hard or uninteresting task. As the example for my child of how to conduct oneself in the world, I fall short in ways that I am perfectly well aware of and I find it disheartening and very very sad," said Vicky, 42, mother of a school-age child.

It's important to do your best. But at the same time, guilt can hamstring us and blind us to the good aspects of our parenting, and it can also prevent us from doing even better. I'd like to liberate my fellow sisters in ADD from this guilt. A tall order! We need to be good parents—but maybe we are effective in our own ways, and we work a little harder in other ways where we have trouble.

▶ FRUSTRATION AND FEELINGS OF INCOMPETENCE

Psychologists talk about a concept of "learned helplessness," which is somewhat parallel to the internalized feelings you may develop as a result of the reactions of others to the symptoms stemming from ADD.

Learned helplessness refers to feelings that result when someone performs tasks for you that you could do for yourself—but these others assume that you can't do. After awhile, you may believe that you can't do them, either. You have learned to be helpless.

SHEDDING A LITTLE LIGHT ON THE SUBJECT

In a study reported in a 1999 issue of *Comprehensive Psychiatry*, researchers reported that women with ADD, particularly those who were primarily impulsive, were much more likely to suffer from seasonal affective disorder (SAD). SAD is an emotional disorder that usually occurs in winter and in areas where the amount of light is significantly decreased. Although the researchers did not also study whether adding light helped women with ADD, since light is effective in helping most SAD sufferers, maybe revving up light levels could be one good solution to try in the dreary days of February.

Said the researchers, "Future studies to assess the effectiveness of light therapy in seasonal ADHD patients would be of great theoretical and practical interest."

Not all moms with ADD have a problem with learned helplessness; however, when a woman has a problem with forgetting things and losing things, others in her family may begin to think that Mom is ineffectual at almost everything. Mom herself may decide that she must be stupid, thus developing a "learned stupid feeling" problem. She knows that she has normal or even above-normal intelligence.

So how come she is doing so many silly things that other people don't have a problem with? In fact, Mom may have been hearing the message for years that she is no good at doing this or that task; and after so long, has begun to accept it. With medication and treatment, however, many children and adults with ADD can be very high performers in many fields of endeavor.

SURROUND YOURSELF WITH POSITIVE PEOPLE

"I think it's important for moms with ADD to try to surround themselves with positive people and, at least when they're little, control the people around your children. My son's Sunday school teachers admire him and his energy," said Juanita, 33, mother of one son.

Knowing that she is not really stupid, the mom with ADD seeks other explanations. She may become very frustrated in her search because, unless you understand the basic problems of ADD, it is very hard to explain why, for example, a smart lady with a Master's degree is constantly losing her car keys or blurting out silly remarks that embarrass her teenagers.

To avoid learned helplessness, challenge the idea that you are incompetent at many or most things. Make a list of what you are good at performing. Think about things you were able to do in the past that you are not doing now. Could you still do those activities if you wished?

Feeling Bad or Defective

Another problem that may occur is that the mom with ADD decides she is somehow defective, or even a bad person. She doesn't know why or how she got to be defective or bad——but there it is. She may also assume, as so many others have assumed for her, that it is her fault. She can't fathom why or how it is her fault, nor does she know how she can be better. "Trying harder" generally hasn't worked very well for her at all.

And once a person internalizes a belief that he or she is bad or stupid, or possibly mentally ill, feelings of self-esteem and overall competency plummet. They may become depressed and avoid other people. They may work in only low-level jobs, afraid to take on harder tasks. They may also wonder where and how they went wrong.

"There's always that little voice in my head that says, 'I should be able to do this, for goodness sakes, I have two college degrees.' I work doubly hard at keeping it together than non-ADD moms. I think I am less patient too. And because of my hypersensitivities, I go crazy when there's too much commotion at home and feel horrible when I see other mothers bask in the insanity of little children who are noisy and running around helter skelter," said Lorraine, 29, mother of two preschoolers.

Lorraine needs to realize that even very smart women can become very frustrated when they are tired and overloaded with responsibilities. She may need more help at home, or she may need to rid herself of some work responsibilities.

Even when a woman is diagnosed with ADD and she has begun treatment, many times vestiges of those old feelings of being bad or stupid can still hang on. They're like sticky, tenacious tar that you can't easily wash off, or even pull off with considerable effort. For this reason, sometimes the woman with ADD can benefit tremendously from consulting with a psychologist or therapist. This topic is covered in more depth in "Professional Help" (Chapter Thirteen).

ARE YOU GETTING ENOUGH SLEEP?

Contrary to popular belief, most adults need at least seven or eight hours of sleep per night. If you are staying up late to talk to your pals in "cyberspace" on the Net, or to catch up on work, or for any other reason, you can develop a serious sleep deficit. As a result, your inattentiveness can become much worse.

Don't let this happen! Get sufficient shut-eye so that you can face the world with enthusiasm—or at least a wide-awake mind—in the morning.

If you find you're having trouble sleeping, whether because of medications or another reason, ask your physician for suggestions on combating insomnia.

Hearing What Others Mean to Say

Sometimes we hear what was said but don't realize what is meant. It's probably easier to illustrate this point by giving you some examples of things people may say to you, what you can *think* that they meant, and possible underlying messages they may want to convey to you.

What Was Said	What You Think Was Meant	What May Have Been Meant
She's a tomboy, just like you were!	She's defective, just like you were	She's full of fun like you were at her age.
What do I know? I'm only your mother	I know everything (unlike you) because I am your mother.	You don't appreciate my advice. You don't listen to me or care what I think.
If my kids acted like that, I would know what to do!	I would beat the tar out of them.	I would remove them from the supermarket.

IT'S OKAY TO CRY SOMETIMES

Sometimes you feel so frustrated, angry, or upset that you just want to cry. But you don't want to be a baby, do you? Isn't it really true that "big girls don't cry"? Nope, it isn't. Sometimes adult women do cry, and the act of crying can release a lot of tension and stress. That's why some people say they are going to have a "good cry." Crying can be therapeutic.

If you're crying or sobbing every day, however, consider that you may be suffering from depression, a problem that doctors report is highly curable.

Lashing Out vs. Listening

Sometimes we moms with ADD overreact to what others say. For example, let's say your sister says if you were *smart*, you'd keep an eye on that teenage son of yours. Instead of jumping to the conclusion, "so you think I am dumb," it's a good idea to find out what she means. Does she know something that you don't know?

Here are sample conversations that start out similarly, but in the first case, the mom with ADD reacts with hostility and in the second case, the mom maintains her cool. Remember, it may not always be important information that your critic has. But it's worth finding out, when it's your child, isn't it?

Conversation One: Adeline Angry and Her Sister Sue

Sue: If you were smart, you would know it's a good idea to be careful with teenagers nowadays.

Adeline: Yeah, yeah. But my son is almost grown and you can't tell them anything anyway, so what's it worth?

Sue: Yes, but sometimes teenagers can get into a lot of trouble really fast.

Adeline: Yes, and sometimes hurricanes happen! So what! I can't do anything about it.

Sue: But what if it was your own son who might be having a problem?

Adeline: Oh, he's fine.

Sue: Well, you might want to check out what he's doing, who he's hanging out with . . .

Adeline: Who are you, the self-appointed police for my family?

Sue: I think you may want to ask your son where he was last night, and who he was with.

Adeline: And I think you should butt out of *my* business and leave *my* family alone! You think you know everything.

Sue leaves and both are very angry.

Conversation Two

Sue: You know, it's a good idea to be careful with teenagers nowadays.

Adeline: Yeah, yeah. But my son is almost grown and you can't tell them anything anyway.

Sue: Yes, but sometimes teenagers can get into a lot of trouble really fast.

Adeline: Like what kind of trouble?

Sue: Hanging out with the wrong people. Sometimes the people closest to you can have some friends you would not approve of.

Adeline: Would you please explain more? I think I'm starting to see where you could be headed, but I'm not sure.

Sue: Well, you might want to check out what your son is doing, whom he's hanging out with . . .

Adeline: Why? Is Tommy hanging out with someone bad?

Sue: I think you may want to ask your son where he was last night, and who he was with.

Adeline: I will ask him. But I'd really appreciate it if you would tell me what you know. Did you see him with someone I wouldn't like? Or did someone tell you this information? I need to know so I can evaluate it better.

Sue: I saw Tommy hanging out with kids a lot older than him, and it looked to me like they were up to no good. I didn't actually see them do anything bad. I just don't like the look of those boys.

Adeline: Thanks for telling me! Where was it, and what were they doing that bothered you? I really need to know.

The conversation continues and Sue tells Adeline everything she knows and why she is worried. They part on good terms.

▶ STRESS

Stress can make almost any problem worse and impair how you do at home and at work. If you are prone to headaches or stomachaches and your stress level is greatly increased, you'll probably get more headaches and stomachaches. The same is true of your ADD symptoms: When you feel overburdened with work and/or family problems, you'll find yourself losing more items, forgetting more things, and other primary ADD symptoms will be exacerbated. For these reasons, it's important to try to keep your stress levels down to a workable level.

Easy for me to say, you might retort! How can you diminish your stress levels in this fast-paced, 21st-century world that we live in? Consider the possibilities described in this section.

Exorcising Stress with Exercise

Who has time to go to the gym? To drive there, change your clothes, and then drive home? If you can't fit formal exercise into your schedule, how about at least one brisk walk a day? Research has revealed that walking is tremendously good for the body: Even walking fifteen to thirty minutes a day can not only improve your body's condition but also enhance your mood.

Here's another idea, since probably no one really likes housework. But if you turn on your favorite music while you vacuum and dust, you may find the chores get done a lot faster and more pleasantly. Vigorous housework can be good exercise.

Riding your bike isn't very hard, and it's also a very positive way to get in shape. Swimming is another pleasurable activity that pays back great dividends in your overall good health.

All of these types of exercise can go far in alleviating the stress and tension that you build up in your daily life.

Cutting Back on Work or Family Responsibilities

You may find that you are working sixty hours a week or more. Is it really worth it? Many people have traded in their high-stress jobs for lower-paying positions that are far more fulfilling. If you can't or are not ready to actually change jobs, perhaps you can work on a "flex time" schedule. Rather than working from 9 to 5, you may find working 6 to 2 or 12 to 8 is a much better fit for your personality and workstyle.

Some people have achieved a good balance at work, but they are drowning in family responsibilities. Some parents seem to feel that all or most of their spare time should go to their children. As a result, Monday it's soccer practice, Tuesday it's piano lessons, Wednesday it's Cub Scouts, and on and on. Try to limit yourself to one major activity per week for each child. The kids may not like it at first. On the other hand, maybe the heavy schedule has been tough on them too!

You thought you were doing them a great favor, but what they really need is some time to play ball with their friends or sit around and read a book. All of us, even our children, need some time to ourselves.

Stopping the Negative Self-Talk

One task that many therapists work on is to help people identify the negative messages they say to themselves—and to actively challenge them. You can discover for yourself what kind of self-talk is going on in your mind, merely by paying attention. For example, if you make a mistake, do you berate yourself as an idiot and tell yourself that you can never do anything right?

Once you identify your negative self-talk, you can challenge it. For example, if you find you belittle yourself when you make a mistake, replace those thoughts with kinder, more positive thoughts: "Okay, I did that wrong. What can I do to avoid this problem in the future?"

Dealing with "System Overload"

The children are fighting again, the soup is boiling over, some guy is at the front door wanting you to sign something, the phone is ringing, you have a report you didn't finish at work that you'll have to write at home tonight, and you feel like you cannot stand another single minute of being in this house with this family. So what do you do?

If you can leave, leave. Get rid of the guy at the front door and deputize your teenager to be in charge for an hour or so. You probably shouldn't drive, because you're so upset that you might crash into someone if you get into that car. Go for a walk at an energetic pace, and go by yourself. When you calm down sufficiently, if you can think of a placid place to go, such as the library, then go there.

If you cannot leave, then count to ten—and do it over and over, *slowly,* if you have to—until you find your rage subsiding to anger. Anger is a negative emotion but it is usually controllable. Rage is a very primitive emotion, and people in the grasp of rage can behave very badly indeed!

Creating a Plan to Deal with the Crisis of Chaos

Psychologist Kathleen Nadeau says one thing you can do is look for triggers and patterns. For example, are there particular times when you are most prone to finding yourself in the midst of a major hissy fit? "I try to identify if there is a trigger, such as you walk in the house from work and see that the kitchen is full of dirty dishes and you start exploding," says Nadeau.

She suggests you do some problem solving. If your children have ADD too, is it realistic to expect them to do the dishes while you're at work? No, it is not. This doesn't mean they shouldn't do them. But it may mean they can do them after you come home, if they've "forgotten" to wash those dishes by now.

Says Nadeau, "It would be much more realistic to establish that, when I get home, it's chore time." She recommends that the mom with this problem would walk in the house, make a cup of tea, and put her feet up. Thus, if a particular time is the trigger, change your routine.

▶ FEARS OF ADD MAKING YOU A BAD MOTHER

Just about anyone feels guilty and expects too much of themselves—but there are so many additional stupid areas for ADD moms to screw up.
—Eileen, 41, a mother of two

Many of the moms I interviewed expressed an intense, underlying fear that their ADD was preventing them from being effective as moms. Or worse, that they were bad mothers because of it—or just bad mothers, for whatever reason. Maybe they weren't trying hard enough.

And yet, isn't this what many women with ADD heard when they were girls? You're not trying hard enough. Whether it was algebra in high school or parenting your child now. Do you feel like you were doing your best then and are still trying now? Maybe it's not the trying-hard part that is a problem.

Said Yvonne, 35, "Before being diagnosed—or even toying with the idea of it, I couldn't understand why I had such difficulty doing things that most people I knew had no trouble with. I equated it to being an incompetent parent. I was constantly battling feelings of guilt over my inability to handle daily tasks like everyone else. Now I realize that my best is all I can give. Most of the time, it's good enough."

Good Moms/Bad Moms: How Can You Tell?

"I was told early on in life that girls just don't have ADD, and later I was told the same about my own daughter. She and I were both labeled negatively, but in different ways. I was a 'bad mother' and she was 'just an unhappy child.' This was the opinion of over 20 professionals throughout my life and my daughter's life. It was also the opinion of relatives, teachers, some friends, and—worst of all—total strangers who thought it was okay to walk right up to me and let me know what they thought of my out-of-control child and my apparent inability to control her," said Denise, 41, and mother of a recently diagnosed 17-year-old daughter.

As discussed in the beginning of this book, society has some very high expectations of moms today, and some of them can be difficult for the mom with ADD to meet. Does this mean that moms with ADD can't be "soccer moms?" Or, worse, does this mean that they will inevitably be bad mothers? Many of the people I interviewed were very worried about that particular issue.

Dealing with the Fear

If traits of ADD are causing parenting problems, then you can work on strategies to resolve them. If it's some vague, indefinable fear of not being good enough, look for specifics. Ask yourself for factual details, including the answers to who, what, when, where, why, and how much.

Here's one strategy you could try. Pretend you are someone else. I'll call her Wendy because I like that name. Wendy is exactly like you, a sort of clone or twin. Now, consider the situation that is troubling you. Or rather, Wendy. Evaluate Wendy as objectively as possible.

Take a particular situation that is troubling, and in your mind, ask Wendy questions like these:

- What was the sequence of events?
- What happened before the problem?
- What did Wendy do when the problem happened?
- What were some of the other choices open to Wendy?
- Why do you think she chose as she did?
- Could she have done things differently or better?
- Did she rectify the situation?
- What was the final outcome?

After you've answered all these questions about Wendy, then you can judge her guilty or not guilty. In many cases, if you can truly depersonalize Wendy and see her as not you but another person, then you can be far more reasonable and objective.

If you still think Wendy really messed up, maybe you are right! Think about what Wendy should do now and should have learned from this experience. But you may also think, hey, Wendy did her best. You give her a not-guilty verdict. Now turn it around. Don't be a harsher critic of yourself than you would be of Wendy.

▶ TRAITS OF BAD MOTHERS

ADHD has not yet been accepted by society as a biological condition and, as a result, ADHD chil-

**dren and their families suffer social conse-
quences and stigma.**
—Associate Professor Judy Kendall in *Family Process*, Spring
1999

If you're wondering whether you're a bad mother, that probably means you aren't one—because most bad mothers really don't care. Often it's the good mothers who are worried about their performance, although it's not healthy to constantly fixate on the goodness or badness of your mothering. I've looked at the abuse issue in depth myself; in 1999, I updated a book called *The Encyclopedia of Child Abuse*.

What Makes a Mother Bad?

During my research, I found many examples of bad/abusive mothers, and I think it would be instructive for readers to take a look at true abusive and neglectful behaviors. Then ask yourself if you exhibit any such behaviors yourself.

Bad Mothers Do These Things

- Beat their children, breaking limbs or causing lasting marks or scars. Some bad mothers actually kill their children. On purpose.
- Leave their children for days or weeks without finding someone else to watch over them.
- Don't take their children to the doctor when they are sick.
- Avoid their children as much as possible.
- Ignore children when they ask for help with a serious problem.
- Refuse to talk to a child's teacher when he or she expresses a concern. Not now and not later.
- Constantly tell the child she or he is stupid and bad. Never notices anything good the child says or does.
- Ignores dangerous behavior. Ignores good behavior.
- Sexually abuses the child or lets someone else sexually abuse him or her.
- Expects behavior beyond a child's capabilities. Expects a one-year-old to be completely potty trained. Expects a four-year-old to watch a baby by herself.
- Forces the child to consume large amounts of substances, such as salt or something unpleasant. One parent forced her child to drink so much water that the child went into seizures and died in the emergency room.

Those are only a few of the many ways that parents can be bad parents. Do you do any of them? If so, you may soon meet social workers at the protective services department in your state. If not, although you may not be perfect and there are undoubtedly areas in which you can improve, you are probably not a bad mom.

What Makes a Mother Good?

How about a list of what good mothers do? I think such a list is a good idea, and so here is mine.

Good Mothers Do These Things

- Love their children.
- Provide food, shelter, and clothing.
- Make sure medical care is provided when a child is sick.
- Take children's feelings into account—but do what's best for the child even if the child doesn't like it. Or even if she hates it.
- Meets the child's friends. If a friend's behavior is problematic and unlikely to change, the good parent may have to prevent her child from seeing that friend.
- Provides a safe environment.
- Is willing to listen to problems and offer suggestions.
- Finds age-appropriate punishments and rewards.
- Apologizes to their child when they are wrong.

▶ COULD IT BE SOMETHING ELSE?

Experts report that a significant number of people with ADD may also have other problems, such as anxiety, depression, and other emotional issues. It may be that the ADD caused the problem, or it may be a separate problem altogether. For example, a person may have both ADD and depression because of a lack of some brain chemical. Or it could be because of two independent processes, or it could even be because of an interaction of various processes. The fact is, you can get a major migraine trying to figure it all out.

What a mom with ADD should primarily be concerned about is not *why* she has ADD, but what she can do about it.

When you have problems with impulsivity, inattentiveness, and sometimes hyperactivity as well, parenting a child can bring moments of frustration and distress. In this chapter, I covered some of the emotions we'd rather not have but do have anyway, such as anger, self-blame, and frustration. Talking about these issues enables moms to understand their feelings—and understanding leads to mastery.

12

Coping with the Holidays and Other Tough Times

What about the really tough times, when you feel that you really can't survive? Other people joke about it, but for me, times like the Christmas holidays are sheer hell.
—Ava, 40, mother of three children

Ava is right—there are some times when parenting and life in general can become an even greater struggle for the ADD mom.

In this chapter I'll concentrate on some of the major difficult times, and offer ideas that have worked for others and may work for you.

- The holidays
- Family celebrations
- Summer vacations
- Traveling
- Sick children

▶ THE HOLIDAYS

One way to make the holidays less stressful is to scale back, while at the same time taking your family's needs and wishes into account. Have a family meeting and make sure everyone comes to it, including your three-year-old.

Tell the family you'd like a simpler holiday, but you want to know what one element or task of the holidays each person feels is really important and that they would feel sad about if you did not do this. For some people, it might be a holiday dinner; for others, it might be caroling in the neighborhood. Others might like the reading of special stories or attending religious ceremonies. You might be very surprised by what you learn from this meeting!

Then incorporate these ideas into your holiday plan. Thus, if you know that one member thinks the midnight church service is the most important thing to do to make the holidays meaningful, then you put that in your plan.

▶ CHILDREN'S BIRTHDAYS OR SPECIAL PARTIES

One of the items on the Ideal Mom list is that she has wonderfully organized birthday parties for her children. The reality, however, for both the non-ADD mom and the mother with ADD, is that most women have little time for planning a lavish and complicated party. However, this does not mean you can't have a party for your child.

Kathleen Nadeau, a noted psychologist and ADD author, says that she knew a successful woman who was planning a party for her son and a few friends, but was obsessing over the homemade lasagna she felt she should prepare. *When* she should do this, she wasn't so sure. Nadeau told her to order a few pizzas or put on a pot of chili—the kids would probably like the pizza or chili much better.

MOMS, DON'T TRY THIS AT HOME!

It's easy for a mom with ADD to get bored or frustrated when she has a houseful of relatives, the meal is finished, and clean-up is over. What you should *not* do is to try to liven up the situation by saying something like, "Gee, what do you think of ____ as candidate for president? I can't stand him!" This is what I did a few years ago at Thanksgiving, and I was amazed at how quickly the overstuffed guests became animated and then angry as they tried to convince each other their political beliefs were wrong. I didn't like the yelling, so I went into another room to watch cartoons with the children. My husband soon found me. "You!" he said. "You started this and then you leave?"

I had to dispense aspirins to at least three guests, who said they had terrible headaches. Lesson learned: If you are having a placid but boring holiday with a houseful of relatives, don't throw out any verbal grenades. Not worth it!

▶ SUMMER VACATIONS FROM SCHOOL

Whether you work outside your home or not, summer vacation from school can be problematic. If you already have your child in a daycare facility, then you may wish to have the child continue attending at the same place. But if your child is age 12 or over, you may find him or her seriously resisting the idea of going to a daycare facility with small children.

For this reason, and if you can afford it, you may wish to send your child to a summer camp, an option available for kids as young as 8 and as old as 17. You can choose from a broad variety of summer camps in the United States, and you can send your child for one or two weeks or for the entire summer. Some camps (a few are listed in Appendix F) specialize in working with children who have ADD. Many camps operate during the day and are run by city or county organizations. Check with your local school as well as city government.

A summer camp for children who have ADD can be a nice break for both your child and for you! Camps generally last at least a week, and a few last all summer long. Prices for camps vary, but expect to pay at least $400–$500 and perhaps more than $1,000, depending on where, how long, and so forth.

One camp, SOAR, is specifically oriented to children with attention deficit disorder. Based in North Carolina, SOAR has camps around the United States and even some in other countries. I don't think it's absolutely necessary that your child with ADD attend a camp that specializes in ADD, but you should make sure that any camp you consider does believe ADD is real and is willing and able to give medication, if your child is taking any medicine.

▶ TRAVEL JOYS AND WOES

Maybe you think you've planned the perfect vacation. You've identified a beautiful site with fun things for both you and your spouse and your children. You've been looking forward to it for weeks or even months. Now the time is here. Will it be as great as you hoped for? Maybe—but watch out for overly exalted expectations. And don't get derailed by common problems that face many families.

Are We There Yet?

Whether you go by car, plane, or boat—or ride a llama to your destination—somehow you have to get there. The trip may be short or long, but time must elapse before you get there. If you can take into account possible problems, the trip itself will be less torturous.

For example, long drives or plane rides are boring to most children, especially when they have ADD. If you can bring a simple game or two and some nutritious snacks such as a few apples, that could help a lot. You also should take "potty breaks" into account when you are driving there yourself. If you are with a person who feels he or she has "failed" unless they drive nonstop for at least five hours, you can have some serious problems with small children.

They nearly always have to go to the bathroom, usually when you are at the most remote site you have ever been in. For this reason, it's good to think ahead and stop every few hours and tell the children to use the toilet. You can allay a lot of disasters this way. Giving your children a chance to stretch their legs and move about can be very rejuvenating as well.

Some people get headaches or stomachaches from long car drives. You may need over-the-counter medication, as well as a few breaks from the car, to deal with this problem.

Surviving an Overnight Visit

Staying overnight in an unknown hotel can be great fun, or a horrible nightmare. The bed feels different, the room may "smell funny" to you, sounds are different, and it can be hard to sleep. Here a few ideas to help the mom with ADD:

- Bring your own pillowcase from home. If you are hypersensitive, as some moms with ADD are, the feel and smell of your pillowcase can really help you relax and get to sleep.
- If your children have ADD, bring their pillowcases too, as well as a small toy that is familiar. Many preschool children like to bring their favorite blanket.
- If you can afford it and your children are school-age or adolescents, get adjoining rooms at a hotel. The kids can watch the programs they like and feel very grown-up. You can have some privacy and a chance to wind down. Your children will pop in and out of your room every five minutes at first, but they'll usually settle down.
- Don't seek the perfect planned vacation or let your spouse rigidly plan every minute. A vacation is a good time to allow yourself some impulsive indulgences—to eat in a restaurant you notice from the highway, stop off in a park you didn't know, or suddenly decide to have a picnic. One year while driving our son to camp, we accidentally discovered Helen, Georgia, on the map, an entire town with a Bavarian theme. Intrigued, we drove there and enjoyed a stay of several days.

Some Dissension Is Normal and Okay

Many times we think, okay, I want this vacation to be just right. I worked hard! I earned it! You want it to be idyllic, just like in the travel brochures. Rather than getting caught up in some imaginary Eden, come back to reality and realize that sometimes kids get sick, people argue, and things aren't just as planned. Use your innate creativity and adaptability to deal with whatever comes up.

▶ WHEN YOUR CHILDREN ARE SICK

When your children suffer from the flu or other ailments, that can be very tough. They're cranky or demanding. Or worse, they just lie there, looking very very sick.

This is a hard time for a mother. It's even harder if you have more than one child, and they're both sick at about the same time. And then you come down with the flu yourself, but you don't really have "time" to be sick.

Obviously, you need to ask your children's physician for help when your kids are sick. You also need to get yourself treated if you become ill. You can't be an effective caregiver when you're crashing around the house with a 103-degree fever yourself.

If your spouse can help you, enlist his help. If your neighbors or family members can provide assistance, take advantage of it. There are also a few places that provide care for mildly sick children. If you are more ill than your child is, you may wish to take advantage of such an opportunity.

I have been sick with "walking pneumonia" while caring for two healthy, active toddlers when my husband was away on a business trip. Here's how I survived, in addition to getting help from others:

- Drink a lot of fluid.
- It's okay if you skip bathing the kids for a few days.
- It's okay if they eat pancakes (or order pizza) for dinner because you're too tired or sick to make something nutritious.
- You don't have to make the beds or do any housework beyond cleaning up serious spills that someone could slip on.
- You should hire a babysitter if you can't stay awake enough to watch small children.

Sometimes you have trouble getting your act together, no matter how hard you try. You may need the help of a physician, psychologist, or therapist. You may also find that medication can help you feel much better. For many people, a support group is what they need. I'll cover these topics in the next chapters.

Even when you feel you have it pretty much all together, when it comes to winter holidays, birthday parties, and traveling with your kids on a trip—the most "together" mom can feel she's falling apart. If you have ADD, you can feel pretty frazzled and pretty fast. In this chapter, I offered some coping strategies.

PART FOUR

Getting Outside Help

Many moms with ADD feel like they're completely alone. But they are not! It's a good idea to realize that there are many other women just like you. A support group may be very helpful. But it may well be insufficient; many women also seek assistance from psychologists or psychiatrists. They need the help that a therapist can provide, and they may also need the medication that only a medical doctor can prescribe.

The next section covers finding professional help and discusses medication for people with ADD. It also describes the kind of help that a support group can offer.

13

Professional Help

Sometimes you may need some extra help from a trained professional. It's okay to ask for help. This chapter provides:

- Self-Test: Do you need therapy?
- Information on medical doctors and how they can help
- Explanation of how psychologists can provide assistance
- Discussion on help provided by social workers and therapists
- Advice on what to do if an expert says you really don't have ADD
- Guidelines on how to find a good professional

There are a variety of "mental health" professionals who can assist you in determining whether you have ADD and, if you do, how to treat it. But first, let's start with a brief self-test to help you consider whether you may need a therapist.

▶ SELF-TEST: SHOULD YOU CONSIDER SEEKING THERAPY?

Answer true or false to each of the following questions.

	True	False
1. I feel like I am stuck in quicksand and starting to sink.		
2. I've been losing many important items, and I just can't find them.		
3. I tend to blurt out what I'm thinking; and lately, it's gotten worse.		
4. I'm very distractible and it's hurting my job. I'm worried I might get fired.		

| | True | False |

5. I went to the supermarket and left the baby in the cart in
the parking lot. I figured this out after I got home.

6. I start to clean my house in one room and pick up something
and head into the next room. Then I go to another room
and get distracted there. It's rare that I get one room
completely done.

7. I feel like I'm not performing as well as I should be at work
or home, mostly because I have trouble paying attention.

There are no specific numbers of "yes" answers that indicate that you should see a therapist, and these questions are offered for guidance only. However, if you answered yes to all or most of them, a therapist might be able to provide you with assistance and advice on some ways to deal with your ADD and the spillover emotions such as feelings of anger, guilt, and other emotions that are often associated with ADD (as discussed in "Coping with Emotions," Chapter Eleven).

▶ MEDICAL DOCTORS: FROM GENERAL PRACTITIONERS TO PSYCHIATRISTS

In many cases of childhood ADD, the child is treated by a pediatrician; however, with adult ADD, the adult is more likely to be treated by a psychiatrist and sometimes by a neurologist. Internists or general practitioners could also diagnose ADD and prescribe medication, but many are reluctant to do so and would prefer to defer to a psychiatrist's diagnosis. In fact, in most cases, it would be better if children were treated by child psychiatrists than by pediatricians, because child psychiatrists have much more training and experience in treating ADD than pediatricians or family practitioners.

What Psychiatrists Do

Psychiatrists are medical doctors who specialize in emotional disorders, ranging from mild to very severe problems such as psychoses. A psychotic person has difficulty distinguishing reality from fantasy and is very dysfunctional, although even the most extreme forms of mental illness can be treated today. Certainly most doctors do not consider ADD even close to extreme, although it can impair a person's life, depending on the severity of the impulsivity, inattention, and/or hyperactivity.

Most people clutch up at the word *psychiatrist*. It has so many scary connotations, like insane asylum, mad doctors doing experiments on people, electroshock therapy, and so forth. Also, if you see a psychiatrist, then you must be crazy, right?

No! Most of the patients psychiatrists see are people with serious life problems and who are diagnosed with depression, ADD, anxiety, and other emotional problems. Very few are psychotic. Most doctors, including psychiatrists, don't like treating severely mentally ill people and much prefer to treat people with less severe emotional disorders.

Psychiatrists can also prescribe medication if you need it. Psychologists, therapists, and social workers cannot prescribe medication because they are not medical doctors. They can only refer you to a doctor if medication is indicated.

If you see a psychiatrist, don't expect her to whip out her prescription pad five minutes after you first meet. Instead, the doctor will want to determine for herself that you really do have ADD. To achieve this, she'll ask you many different questions. Some doctors may also wish to contact others such as parents or your siblings—with your permission—in an attempt to determine if you had any symptoms of ADD as a child.

An accurate diagnosis is very important, and psychiatrists realize this. Some people may think that they have ADD and they may instead have another problem. They may also have an underlying medical problem; for example, hyperthyroidism might mimic hyperactivity. The treatment for an overactive thyroid gland is very different from the treatment for ADD.

The doctor will also try to determine if you could have other problems in addition to ADD; for example, many people with ADD may have some degree of depression. Others may have a problem with anxiety.

After the doctor diagnoses you—which may take several sessions, depending on the physician—she will decide if medication might help you. Then the doctor will need to choose which medication you should take. Most doctors realize that people with ADD should take medication as infrequently as possible, such as once or twice a day, because many have trouble remembering to take the medicine. The doctor will also consider what other medications you are taking now to make sure that there won't be a problem with "mixing" the medicines, and that you won't have any side effects resulting from a bad drug interaction.

In general, the doctor will try the lowest possible efficacious dose to see if it has any impact and may decide to increase the dosage as treatment continues. Psychiatrists monitor your response to medication, and they will either change the dosage or the medication itself if it isn't helping you. Read "Medications That May Help" (Chapter Fourteen) for more information.

Screening Doctors

The way many people find a psychiatrist is to look in the Yellow Pages or at an HMO or managed care listing and pick the doctor nearest to where they live. You might think that calling the local medical society would be a good idea, but many doctors advise against this strategy as well. The medical society is likely to give you doctors who aren't very busy and who happen to be members of their organization.

Instead, try the following tactics to locate a physician, who you should then screen:

1. **Ask local chapters of national organizations.** You can contact national organizations to find out where local chapters are, and then you can call the president or leader of those groups to find out who is treating ADD. If the leader doesn't want to tell you over the phone, attend a few meetings of the group.

CHADD (Children and Adults with Attention Deficit Disorder) in Washington and the National Alliance for the Mentally Ill (NAMI) are both listed in Appendix C. I don't consider ADD to be a "mental illness," but I do know that ADD is one issue that NAMI has covered in the past. You could ask the national office of NAMI for the name of the chapter nearest to you and a phone number that you can call.

2. **Ask medical schools, if nearby.** If there are any medical schools within a hundred-mile radius of where you live, I would contact them for possible referrals. They may have graduates who reside in your area. Contact the psychiatry department or write them a letter.

Meeting with the Doctor

You can't really know if you will be able to trust and to establish a rapport with the doctor until you meet him or her. You may be able to talk to the doctor on the phone, but often you will not because they are so busy. In general, you'll need to make an appointment to meet the doctor.

If the psychiatrist tells you that you should have a physical examination with your regular doctor before he sees you, then get one. In fact, get one anyway, even if no one does suggest it to you. If you have a medical problem such as thyroid disease, it could mimic the hyperactivity found in ADD. Other conditions might resemble ADD. But treating you with Ritalin or psychotherapy won't help when your problem is not ADD.

When you do meet a new doctor, be sure to ask questions. Here is a list to tailor and adapt to your own needs.

1. **Do you think attention deficit disorder is real?** If the doctor tells you that ADD is just a passing fad—and you feel strongly that ADD is probably your problem—then clearly, this physician is not the right one for you. You don't need to ask any more questions. You're done. Move on.

2. **Do you think that women can have ADD?** The doctor may believe that ADD is a problem—but for boys. If he hasn't updated his knowledge to realize that many women can and do have ADD, then he is the wrong doctor for you. Next!

3. **Have you treated people with ADD before?** In most cases, it's best to work with a physician who is experienced with your particular problem. Thus, even if the doctor thinks ADD is a valid diagnosis and even if he thinks that, yes, women can have ADD, if he has no professional experience, this can be a negative point

against him. However, you may still consider him, especially if there are few or no other doctors near your home. All the better if he says that he is willing and eager to learn everything he can about ADD and the best treatments.

4. **Do you believe that medication can help a person with ADD?** This one isn't a clear-cut "right" or "wrong" answer. Although I believe that medication is generally what is needed by a person with ADD, if you are strongly opposed to medication, then this is a good question to ask the doctor. However, most psychiatrists and other medical doctors do believe that medication is important. If you are opposed to taking medication, maybe you should start with a psychologist or therapist and skip the medical doctor altogether.

5. **Should therapy with a psychologist or other person supplement medical treatment?** This is another question that doesn't have a right or wrong answer but is really dependent on what you want. Many doctors do believe that it's important to supplement medication with therapy, but they may not provide the therapy "part." In that case, you would need to see someone else. If you want to see only one person, you would need a psychiatrist who isn't adamant about your seeing a therapist too.

6. **How frequently do you see new patients, in general?** Doctors are usually quite resistant about telling you how many times they will need to see you, but it's still an important question to ask. If you happen to see one of the rare physicians who still practice psychoanalysis only (a form of therapy requiring very intensive, long-term treatment), then he may say you will need to see him several times a week or even more frequently.

In most cases, and unless your problems are life threatening, the doctor can see you once a week or less frequently, and that will be enough.

7. **If you treat me and I improve, about how often would I need to see you after that?** This is a good question to ask because if you are improving, then you should generally be seeing the doctor less frequently. However, if you are still taking medication, you should see the doctor at least once every three to six months.

WHO HAS WHAT DEGREES?

Psychiatrist: Medical Doctor

Psychologist: Ph.D. in Psychology

Therapist: Master's in Counseling

Social Worker: Master's in Social Work

► PSYCHOLOGISTS: WHAT THEY CAN AND CANNOT DO

A psychologist is a person with a Ph.D. in psychology or counseling and who is licensed by the state to provide psychological counseling. A psychologist may practice alone or in a group with other psychologists and sometimes in a group with psychiatrists too.

How Can a Psychologist Help?

A psychologist experienced with patients with ADD can diagnose a person with ADD and can also provide counseling. As mentioned earlier, they cannot prescribe medication, although the psychologist may think that medication would help and may refer you to a psychiatrist.

Often adults with ADD need the counseling help that a good psychologist can provide. The mom with ADD may have a problem with low self-esteem or with feeling incompetent at parenting and other aspects of her life. The psychologist can train you to consider your own negative "self-talk", for example, when you make a mistake, saying in your mind, "I'm so stupid! I can't do anything right!" A psychologist will help a person challenge such thoughts.

Psychologists (and therapists) can also provide help to a mom in dealing with the negative emotions discussed in "Coping with Emotions" (Chapter Eleven), such as guilt and anger as well as other emotions.

There are many different kinds of therapy, but many psychologists use "cognitive-behavioral" therapy, which basically means that the psychologist helps you rethink how you think about yourself, assists you in challenging maladaptive ideas, and helps you change your behavior. However, some psychologists rely on other forms of therapy that may be ineffectual for the person with ADD.

How Should You Screen Psychologists?

In general, you can use the same techniques used to screen doctors when you are screening psychologists, including asking people at local chapters of national organizations such as CHADD and NAMI. You could also contact the head of the psychology department of the nearest university to see if there are any practicing psychologists that he or she would recommend.

You should also meet with the psychologist before deciding to work with her or him. Many but not all psychologists are willing to talk with you briefly on the phone for no charge. Still, you can't really make up your mind until you meet. You should be sure to have questions ready to ask, including questions similar to what you would ask a psychiatrist. Again, some questions might include

- Do you think attention deficit disorder is real?
- Do you think that women can have ADD?

- Have you treated people with ADD before?
- Do you believe that medication can help a person with ADD?
- How often do you see new patients, in general?
- If you treat me and I show improvement, about how often would I need to see you after that?

I think these questions are self-explanatory, with one exception. I would ask the psychologist if he or she believes medication is important, because this is a critical issue in ADD. If your doctor wishes to treat you with Ritalin but a psychologist thinks that all ADD medications are bad, then you have a conflict that would need to be resolved.

If you are opposed to medication, you may choose a different doctor or decide not to see a psychiatrist at all. But if you do believe medication might help you, and the psychologist is opposed to ADD medications, then you need a different psychologist.

Others Who Treat Adults with ADD: Social Workers and Therapists

Therapists and social workers are also often interested in ADD and can provide counseling and practical advice. A therapist may have a master's degree in counseling or psychology and may be licensed by the state to provide therapy. A social worker has a degree in social work, preferably an MSW (master's in social work) and is licensed to provide counseling.

The professional license given by credentialing organizations, as well as by the state licensing board to therapists (or medical doctors or psychologists), authorizes the person to treat individuals. But keep in mind that having a license is no insurance that these professionals are skilled at what they do, nor does it imply that they have expertise in particular areas such as ADD.

You should be sure to meet with the social worker or therapist before making any long-term commitments with this person. In general, you could ask him or her the same questions you would ask the psychologist.

▶ WHAT IF THE "EXPERT" SAYS YOU DON'T HAVE ADD?

Sometimes people are absolutely convinced that they have attention deficit disorder. After all, they sometimes lose things and are somewhat impatient. But the point is, how severe are the symptoms and how disruptive to your life are they? If losing or forgetting problems are really disrupting your life, you may have ADD. You may also have another problem, such as depression or anxiety disorder. The doctor may be right.

Then again, the doctor may be wrong. How could a physician make a diagnostic mistake? There are several reasons for failing to diagnose ADD in a woman:

- The doctor has little or no experience in treating ADD.
- The doctor doesn't think ADD is a valid diagnosis—to him, it isn't "real."
- The doctor specializes in depression, anxiety disorders, or another problem and tends to "see" this disorder in many of his patients.
- You may be primarily inattentive rather than hyperactive.
- The doctor thinks only boys and men can have ADD.

My first two points are self-explanatory, but let me further explain the other items in my list.

1. **The doctor specializes in depression, anxiety disorders, or other problems** If most of the doctor's patients suffer from depression or anxiety, he may "see" depression or anxiety in you. In fact, you may *be* depressed or anxious—but the root cause could be ADD. Even physicians who treat ADD sometimes admit that they too can see ADD in everyone and must be careful to pay close attention to symptoms because the problem may be something else altogether.

2. **You may be primarily inattentive rather than hyperactive.** If the doctor perceives that it isn't "real" ADD unless the person is bouncing off walls, and you are not hyperactive, then he may refuse to diagnose you with ADD.

3. **The doctor thinks only boys and men can have ADD.** There are still many psychiatrists and psychologists who see ADD as a male problem and, if they do believe that some girls and women may have ADD, think that they are extremely rare indeed.

▶ FINDING A GOOD PROFESSIONAL

Here are some ways to find a good psychiatrist, psychologist, or therapist:

- Ask your doctor.
- Ask your clergyperson.
- Ask someone you know who is seeing a therapist.

There's still a certain stigma attached to seeing a psychiatrist, psychologist, or therapist. But whether it's because we don't want to be seen as "crazy," or we think we should be strong, independent women who pull ourselves up by our bootstraps, the fact is that mental health professionals can help a mom with ADD in many ways. A qualified expert who is experienced and knowledgable about ADD can diagnose you and treat you and also provide practical advice. In this chapter I covered the role of psychiatrists, psychologists, and therapists and discussed how to find one.

14

Medications That May Help

**The meds stop me from spinning. Spinning is
my own term to describe myself when I'm trying to do eight different things at one time and
not able to start anything at all. After taking
my meds, I can say to myself "Stop!" on whatever is not working.**
—Anita, 38, mother of one 12-year-old boy

Many moms with ADD—although not all—take medication to help them concentrate and focus better and to control other symptoms of ADD such as impulsivity,
inattentiveness, and so forth. Medicine won't solve all your problems, but it may
be able to give you an extra "edge" or a boost up, so that you now find that you
can scale a mental wall that you were unable to climb before. Some women eschew
prescribed medications and instead rely on herbal remedies such as ginkgo biloba,
mineral supplements, or other choices. Or they try altering their diet.

In this chapter, I'll focus on the following information and issues involved in taking medication as part of your ADD treatment:

- Dealing with your fear of taking "drugs"
- Taking ADD-specific medications
- Considering other medications
- Learning how doctors select ADD medications
- Looking at the pros and cons of taking medication
- Knowing if the medicine is working
- Trying "natural" or alternative remedies
- Making changes in your diet
- Using homeopathy and biofeedback

If you think you may need medication for ADD, be sure to rely upon the advice of your own medical doctor. This chapter is provided as an overview for general educational purposes only, and in no way should the information here be construed as medical advice.

▶ **FEAR OF TAKING "DRUGS"**

It is true that some people abuse stimulant medications. As a result, these medications are carefully controlled by the Food and Drug Administration (FDA). It's also true that many insurance companies restrict patients to receiving only thirty days of a medication at a time.

Partly because the FDA heavily controls these medications, some people think that they will be seen as "druggies" if they take such medications. If you feel your pharmacist is treating you negatively or unfairly, then you should change pharmacies. You should also complain about the pharmacist to the store manager.

DOES MEDICATION HELP?

Moms with ADD whom I interviewed said:

- I am calmer, more deliberate in my actions. I think more linearly and the chaos in my head is minimized. I don't feel quite so anxious and emotional.

- The zoning out was cut by about 85 percent. I exhaust myself much less from the effort to concentrate, and I screw up much less. The foggy feeling went away.

- I have much less difficulty with patience, staying on task, remembering things long term (like appointments). Before the meds, I hated working, got tired easily and bored quickly, never stayed with anything, never finished anything. I now have a job and look forward to climbing to higher levels.

- The medicine helps me concentrate and calms down my hyperactivity.

- I am better able to focus on projects to see them through to completion.

- There is far less "noise" in my mind.

- They give me more control over my thought processes. I am less distractible, less frustrated, and therefore less irritable. I can cope with interruptions and distractions without totally losing track of where I was.

- I now can participate in conversations without blinking out and can retrieve information in my head when asked a question.

- For the first time, I can actually set goals and have an idea how to get from point A to point B to achieve them.

In addition to adult worries about taking ADD medications, often parents worry about giving stimulants to their children and fear this could lead to taking illegal drugs such as cocaine. Researchers have actually found the reverse to be true.

A 1999 study of teenage boys diagnosed with ADD found that boys who had been receiving medication for ADD had an 84 percent *decrease* in the use of substances such as cocaine, alcohol, marijuana, hallucinogenic drugs, and a variety of stimulants. Said Alan I. Leshner, of the National Institute on Drug Abuse (NIDA), "Treating the underlying disorder, even if with stimulants, significantly reduces the probability they [children] will use drugs later on."

Keep in mind that new medications are introduced all the time, including new formulations; for example, a transdermal Ritalin patch may be released in 2000 or 2001. Such a patch would alleviate the problem of forgetting to take your medication.

CAN ADD MEDICATIONS PREVENT LATER SUBSTANCE ABUSE?

In a study report released in 1999, funded by the National Institute on Drug Abuse and the National Institute of Mental Health, researchers reported that teenage boys who had been receiving medications for attention deficit hyperactivity disorder were much *less* likely to abuse alcohol, cocaine, marijuana, and other substances when they became teenagers.

The researchers at Massachusetts General Hospital, Harvard School of Public Health, and Harvard Medical School compared substance abuse disorders in 56 boys with ADHD who had been receiving medication for about four years to boys with ADHD who had not been treated with any stimulant medications. Researchers also compared both groups to boys who did not have ADD.

The study revealed that 75 percent of the ADD boys who had not received medication had a substance disorder problem with one or more substances. This finding contrasted sharply with the boys with ADD who had received medication: 25 percent of them had developed a substance abuse disorder. As for the boys who did not have ADD, 18 percent had developed a problem. As a result, medication apparently had a very positive impact on the boys with ADD who received it. Although they had a higher rate (25%) of substance abuse problems than the non-ADD boys (18%) did, it was drastically lower than the nonmedicated boys with ADD.

Said NIDA Director Alan I. Leshner, "While some clinicians have expressed concern about giving stimulants to children with ADHD because they fear it might increase the risk that these children will abuse stimulants and other drugs when they get older, this study shows exactly the opposite."

▶ ADD-SPECIFIC MEDICATIONS

There are specific medications that most physicians use to help children and adults diagnosed with ADD. The medications of choice fall into the stimulant class and include such medications as Ritalin (methylphenidate), Dexedrine (dextroamphetamine) or DexroStat, Adderall or Cylert (pemoline), and Desoxyn (methampethamine).

There are also medications that fall into other categories, such as antidepressants, that may be used to help a child or adult with ADD.

When these medications "work," they enable individuals to think more clearly, focus on tasks longer, and they also work to aid in control of other ADD symptoms. Some studies have noted that children who don't have ADD can also focus better when they take stimulants. Does that mean everyone should take stimulants? No, it does not. If a child does not have ADD, then in most cases he or she can sufficiently focus on tasks, while the child with ADD struggles to focus. What comes naturally to the non-ADD child or adult is not innate to the child or adult with ADD. The stimulants, when they help the person with ADD, can give them a boost to function more like a non-ADD person.

▶ OTHER MEDICATIONS

There are other medicines that can help many people with ADD even though they are not specifically chosen for ADD. For example, some antidepressants may be very helpful to individuals with ADD. This doesn't necessarily mean that if they work, you must have been depressed (although you could have been). The fact is that doctors prescribe antidepressants for many uses, including as a mild painkiller for chronic pain. Do *ask* your doctor, however, if you are concerned that the physician may be diagnosing you with depression but for some reason is not telling you so.

Antidepressant Medications

Most people have heard of Prozac (fluoxetine), which is one very popular antidepressant. But there are many others. There are different categories of antidepressants, such as tricyclics and *selective serotonin reuptake inhibitors,* or SSRIs for short. Desipramine is an example of a tricyclic, while Prozac is an example of an SSRI. Some women may find SSRIs increase their problems with dreaminess and forgetfulness.

If the doctor prescribes a drug from one category of antidepressants, such as one in the tricyclics category, and that doesn't help the patient, the doctor may decide to try a medication from a different category, assuming that another tricyclic probably wouldn't help you either.

Some of the newer antidepressants, such as Wellbutrin (buproprion), may help people with depression or with ADD. And if the person has both ADD and depression, the doctor may feel such a medication might be indicated.

Combinations of Medications

Sometimes physicians choose to combine several medications to treat ADD more effectively. For example, the doctor may prescribe an antidepressant and a stimulant medication. Another reason they may prescribe several medications is that a person could have both ADD and anxiety or both ADD and depression. There is considerable overlap between ADD and such disorders.

▶ HOW DOCTORS SELECT MEDICATIONS FOR ADD

Many people are surprised to learn that doctors often must adjust psychiatric medications over time, rather than knowing right away the exact dosage every person needs. However, many medications for ADD aren't strictly calibrated to body weight or other parameters, and there's an art to choosing the right medication and the right dosage.

The fact is that medications for emotional issues are very different from the antibiotic you take for a strep throat or a bladder infection. In those cases, the doctor knows you have an infection because he has a lab test that tells him so.

If he did a culture of the bacteria, the lab would inform him what medicine killed the bacteria, and he could then prescribe the right medication with great confidence. He also can use factors such as your weight to consider what dosage of medication to give you and decide how frequently you should take the medication. (And in the case of a person with ADD, it should be as simple a regimen as possible, to eliminate opportunities to forget to take the medicine!)

But when it comes to ADD, the doctor can't order a lab test to definitively prove that you "have" it—because there aren't any such lab tests. There are some fancy x-rays that may indicate the existence of ADD. But try and convince your insurance company to pay for them. As a result, the doctor will base the diagnosis primarily on how you present now, your past history, and his own judgment.

As a result, the doctor will prescribe the medication that he feels has the best chance to work for you. He'll also expect to see you back within the timeframe he recommends, so you can report on how you feel and any side effects that you may have experienced.

Your physician must also take into account that some medications have a cumulative effect and build up in your system. This means that they often don't work dramatically in the beginning; but instead, you may see improvement weeks or even months later.

The fact is that there is plenty of art as well as science involved for the physician who is determining the medications to prescribe for individuals with ADD, depression, and other emotional issues. This is why you need a doctor who is very knowledgeable about ADD. In most cases, that person is a psychiatrist or sometimes a neurologist rather than your internist or other physician.

▶ PROS AND CONS OF MEDICATION

Before any medication enters your mouth, you should first consider the pros and cons of taking medication for your ADD. Many medications can be very helpful in decreasing symptoms; however, it is also true that they may cause side effects that are troublesome for you.

The Benefits of Medication

When your medication works, you will find a reduction in your ADD symptoms. It will be easier to remember things and to focus on what you want to zero in on, rather than whatever subject your mind wanders off to. You'll still need to issue periodic reminders to yourself to do this or that—but you will listen better to yourself.

Some people say that their medication enabled them, for the first time in their lives, to feel really aware of what was going on all around them. At last, they felt they could truly focus.

The Down Side

There are negative aspects to every medication. Following are the two primary "cons" to taking medicine for your ADD:

Taking Your Medication on Time
The drug regimen may be too hard for you. If you can't remember to take a medication three or four times a day, ask the doctor if the drug comes in a sustained-release form that you can take less frequently.

Medication "compliance" (taking your medicine) is a big problem for many people and especially so when you have ADD. It's not so much that the ADD mom doesn't want to take her medicine: She simply forgets. Here are some ways to remember:

- Use a watch, clock, pager, or other device that alerts you to take your medicine.
- Find out if there is a sustained-release form of the medication that you take. This would mean you would get the same effect but could take the medicine fewer times per day.
- Link medicine to another event, such as breakfast or another meal. Or before you do another task that you know you will do, such as brushing your teeth.
- Placing the medicine in a site where you can't miss it (such as next to your toothbrush).
- Attach your pillbox to your toothbrush with a rubber band.

- If you take more than one pill, keep the medications together.
- Use a pillbox in which you put in your medicine days ahead of time. If, for example, "Monday" is empty, then that means you took the medicine on Monday. Of course, you must remember to put the medicine in the pillbox in the first place.

Dealing with Side Effects

Your side effects may be too problematic. When considering side effects, keep in mind that anything, even water, if taken in excess, can make you sick. If the side effects to a medicine are too severe, then you will probably need to stop taking it and find another medication that works for you better.

Here is a list of some of the side effects that medication can sometimes cause. This list is not medication-specific, and you should consider the side effects of the particular drug you are taking. For example, there is a risk of seizures in taking higher doses of Wellbutrin, and that risk is lower with other medications.

- Diarrhea
- Heart palpitations
- Dizziness
- Stomach pain or heartburn
- Decreased sexual drive

Sometimes symptoms are mild and abate, and sometimes they are more serious—and abate. It's very important to talk with your doctor about what to watch out for and under what conditions you should stop taking the medicine and call her.

▶ HOW DO YOU KNOW IF THE MEDICINE IS WORKING?

Hopefully, the very first medication the physician prescribes will be the ideal one for you, and you will never need to switch. However, sometimes you will find the initial prescription doesn't really help you, or has side effects that are too troublesome, and thus the doctor must change the medication until she finds a better match between patient and medication.

Some medications take time to work, and you won't feel their full impact for days or even weeks. In addition, some medications may give you a few side effects at first that go away after several days as your body gets used to the new medicine. So, try to give at least a few days' trial of the medication before you give up on it (this is true of many medications, not just drugs for ADD). *Important note:* The exception is when you develop a rash. In that case, call your doctor immediately.

Before you even start taking medicine, it's a good idea to make a list of your ADD symptoms that are most bothersome to you. Be as specific as possible.

Making a List and Checking It Twice

Your list may include such symptoms as restlessness, interrupting other people while they talk, not listening to others, and any of a myriad of symptoms/problems. The more you tailor the list to YOU, the better able you will be to see if the medicine is helping you.

Whenever possible, also be sure to quantify the symptoms. For example, let's say one annoying problem that you have experienced is major anger whenever you have to stop for a red light—you're impatient to get through all of them and on your way to wherever.

After the medication kicks in, you may improve to the point that you will still feel impatient, but only at half the red lights. Or none of them! Such targeted symptoms are called "behavioral markers."

Maybe one of your biggest problems is that you lose too many things. Write down how many times a day you misplace items.

Don't rush making this checklist: Put some thought into it. Think carefully about the problems that you are encountering. Ask your husband or significant other and your children for help—they may have some very good ideas.

Then adapt the checklist to your own needs. Track your behavior for a week or at least a few days. One day is just not enough. It could have been a very bad day or an unusually good one. You need more data to really tell.

I provided a sample chart here, but purposely did not fill it in (I've labeled it "Sally's Specific Symptoms"). I want you to compare yourself to you before medication and you after medication.

A few rules for creating your own checklist:

- Keep it simple! Use only two or three target behaviors as a basis for comparison. It's too confusing if you use more. Later on, if you wish, you can drop some behaviors and add new ones.
- Use the chart *before* you start taking the medicine. Sometimes, the mere fact that you are paying attention to a behavior means that you will modify it. If you check yourself before you initiate medication, you can create a baseline on yourself.
- If you find that your behaviors improve just by paying attention to them, even before you take the medication, consider whether these should be your target behaviors.
- List behaviors that probably stem from ADD, such as behaviors that are impulsive, hyperactive, inattentive, and so forth. Don't expect ADD medication to whiten your teeth or help you find true love.
- If you're not sure if a behavior is ADD-related, ask your doctor or therapist.
- Don't be discouraged if you use the chart and don't see much difference from before and after medicine. If the first medication isn't helping, the doctor can try others.

Sally's Specific Symptoms Checklist

Ritalin (or other name of drug) Start Date: Monday, Oct. 11

	Mon.	Tues.	Weds.	Thurs.	Fri.	Sat.	Sun
I lose 1–2 things per day. Put a "Y" for "yes, I lost something," for each day items were lost. Put an "N" for "not lost" for each day you didn't lose things.							
I am late for work several times a day. Put a "Y" for "Yes, I was late," and an "N" for "No, I was not late."							
I forgot to check Billy's homework. "Y" is "Yes, I forgot." "N" for "No, I did not forget.							

Analyzing Your Lists

When the week is over, go back and compare your pre-medication chart to your post-medication chart. Did any of the targeted behaviors improve, showing more "N's" than before, when you weren't taking the ADD medication? If so, this is good! However, don't expect too much. We're looking for improvement here, not perfection. So you did not "fail" if you find that you still have a few "Y's" remaining on your chart.

Save your first week's chart and repeat the chart for at least several more weeks, so you can track whether you are staying the same or improving. You might also find that there are a few more "Y's" in later weeks. This doesn't necessarily mean that you are failing on this medication. Everyone has ups and downs. But if the medicine is helping, you should notice eventual improvement over your baseline scores before you started the medication.

If you are not satisfied with your progress and you've given the medicine a sufficient trial for at least a month or another timeframe your doctor recommends—and you are being realistic in your expectations—then you may want to ask your physician if you can try a different medication. Save your charts because you can compare yourself on med A versus med B.

▶ "NATURAL" OR ALTERNATIVE MEDICINES

The field of alternative remedies has gone largely unstudied in clinical studies, so it's difficult to say whether certain "health food" drugs can improve your ADD. Many doctors are extremely skeptical of alternative remedies, for this very reason—no studies. Another reason why physicians worry about alternative medicine is that the FDA does not regulate such drugs. The ibuprofen you take for a headache is very strictly regulated; the melatonin you might take for insomnia is not.

This is because Congress passed the Dietary Supplement Health and Education Act of 1994, which was implemented in 1997. This law allowed stores to sell "dietary supplements" that are vitamins, minerals, herbs, amino acids, and other products, the kind of items sold in a "health food" store.

In the case of these products, it is up to the *government* to *prove* a product is unsafe. This is the direct opposite of the case for over-the-counter medicines or prescribed medications. In those cases, the pharmaceutical company must prove to the government first that the product is safe, before they can ever sell it. They must test the medication in clinical studies under controlled conditions. Such studies are not required with health food medications: They can be very expensive, so they are rarely done. My advice is "caveat emptor": Let the buyer beware.

Do Alternative Medicines Work?

My daughter and I take valerian root. Some people take it for insomnia, but we are not tired people. Instead, Valerian slows down our brains, allowing us to focus on one thing at a time.
—Luisa, 42, mother of a 14-year-old girl

Many people have found that alternative medicine has helped them improve their lives. A few studies have indicated improvements with magnesium supplements or zinc supplements; however, this does not mean you should rush out and buy magnesium or zinc for you or your children. Nor should you rely on megavitamin therapy unless your physician recommends it. One study showed that megavitamins increased disruptive behavior by 25 percent among children. Some also had elevated liver enzymes.

It is possible that a microdeficiency of vitamins or minerals is a problem for some people with ADD. Most experts see no problem with taking a daily dose of a multivitamin pill, as long as you follow the instructions. Don't assume "more is better."

Some Things to Consider

Here are a few cautions for those taking alternative medications:

- Just because you bought it in a health food store doesn't mean it's healthy for you.
- An alternative medication (herb, mineral, or any other preparation) is also a drug. It can have side effects.
- Do *not* exceed the dosage recommended on the bottle. *More* is *not* better.
- Tell your doctor you are taking the medication(s). Sure, he may disapprove. He may also tell you that the medication is dangerous because of other health problems you have. Your doctor needs to know all the medications you are taking, whether they are prescribed, over-the-counter, or alternative medicines.

▶ DIETARY CHANGES

About thirty years ago, the "Feingold Diet" was popular among parents of children with ADD, although no scientific evidence supported it then or now. The theory was that an extremely careful diet that avoided food additives and other items the proponents considered harmful could control ADD. Another common fear was that sugar was "making" children hyperactive: This too has been discounted by scientific studies.

Does this mean that diet has no effect whatsoever on people with ADD? We can't rule out diet as important, although I can't offer you the one diet that will eradicate the symptoms of you or your children.

Some studies have shown improvement in some children placed on an elimination diet, which excluded foods that some people are allergic to, such as wheat, corn, peanuts, milk, and others.

According to Anna Baumgaertel, M.D., in her article on alternative and controversial treatments for ADD in a 1999 issue of *Pediatric Clinics of North America,*

Based on the research of the last 20 years, it is difficult to dismiss summarily the findings that a subgroup of children with ADHD responds favorably to individualized elimination diets. A role for behavioral food sensitivity has been defined more clearly. Several specific conclusions can be drawn from this newer research: (1) behavioral improvement is more likely with appropriate elimination diets in individuals with atopic histories [histories of allergies such as asthma], family history of migraine, and a family history of food reactivity; younger children also seem to be more responsive; (2) whole foods as well as additives are implicated, including the common dietary allergens such as milk, nuts, wheat, fish, and soy; (3) because a wide range of behaviors may be responsive to dietary manipulation, specific target behaviors should be elicited from parents and other caretakers, including sleep and mood disturbances in addition to typical ADHD symptoms.

▶ HOMEOPATHY AND BIOFEEDBACK

Homeopathy

Homeopathic remedies are very popular in Europe; however, most medical doctors are wary of homeopathy. The basic principle behind homeopathy is that if you take a tiny dose of a substance that would normally be bad for you, it could then somehow help you. As a result, some migraine preparations include tiny doses of normally deadly substances such as belladonna (deadly nightshade) or other substances.

Most support has come from anecdotal evidence, although one study in Europe illustrated an improvement in ADHD with homeopathic treatment. For now, however, the jury is still out.

Biofeedback

Some studies have indicated that children with ADD can learn to control their skin temperature, pulse rate, and so forth with biofeedback training; however, these children improved neither their behavior nor their ADD symptoms. Experts say that further studies may be indicated. Perhaps biofeedback would work better with adults who have ADD. We need studies in order to know.

Many people diagnosed with ADD fear taking medication and see it as somehow illicit. Yet medication can help many moms with ADD gain some or a great deal of control over their symptoms. In this chapter, I covered the pros and cons of medication, types of medicines given to ADD, and how to determine if medication is helping you.

15

Support Groups, Coaches and Other Forms of Help for the Mom with ADD

I think it's important for moms with ADD to create a network of support, especially with other people who have ADD kids or who are diagnosed with ADD themselves. Most parents of non-ADD kids and non-ADD adults just don't understand it at all. Instead, they are tour guides for guilt trips!
—Sara, 41, mother of two children

In this chapter, I will describe various kinds of support systems for moms with ADD:

- Professional organizers
- ADD coaches
- Support groups and how they can help

▶ PROFESSIONAL ORGANIZERS

This concept can be sort of hard to wrap your mind around if you are a woman with ADD—but the fact is that there are people who earn their entire livings by helping other people organize their homes and offices. They can come into your home and help you figure out what stays and what goes and how to arrange the remaining items that are definite "keepers." They can also offer advice over the phone. Many organizers work with adults, but some also help children.

There is even an organization for such experts: the National Association of Professional Organizers (see Appendix E for more information).

▶ ADD COACHES

An ADD coach is someone you can contract with to advise you weekly on a variety of matters. If your coach is available locally (most are not), he or she may come over to your house and talk with you one-on-one. If a coach is not available locally, you may receive your coaching in a phone conversation, perhaps punctuated by periodic electronic messages if you also have access to a computer.

KATE KELLY: ADD COACH WHO PROVIDES REFERRALS

Kate Kelly, author of *You Mean I'm Not Lazy, Stupid, or Crazy?!* is an ADD coach, and she also offers referrals. Kelly says you can contact her by e-mail at KKDancit@aol.com for further information. As of this writing, she charges about $250 a month. "If you have a particular issue that needs to be discussed in between sessions, I want to hear about it," says Kelly. You may also go to her website at www.addcoaching.com.

Coaching is not considered the same as therapy. Instead of trying to find the roots of conflicts and dealing with deep-seated problems that may exist, coaches offer hands-on, practical advice for solving specific problems and helping you identify stumbling blocks to achieving your goals. The experience and education of coaches vary and may or may not include extensive training. Coaching is not free, although you may be able to obtain reduced rates through contacts with the Optimal Functioning Institute. Contact the Institute through its website at www.addcoach.com.

▶ SUPPORT GROUPS: WHAT THEY ARE AND CAN DO

A support group is an organization of people who are interested in and/or concerned about a particular issue. There are hundreds of support groups nationwide for a rather amazing array of different needs, ranging from groups for alcoholics to groups for people who are afraid of lightning, people distressed by the death of a pet, and so on. Not surprisingly, there are also groups for adults who have ADD.

Sometimes these groups are stand-alone organizations for adults with ADD; other times, they are a subgroup of a national organization called CHADD (Children and Adults with Attention Deficit Disorder). Moms with ADD can usually gain a great deal of knowledge and moral support from either type of group.

CHADD also offers a national conference every year that is well attended by parents of children with ADD, adults with ADD, and professionals. I have attended several conferences and found them to be not only informative but enormously stimulating and fun. Many people at the conference talk very fast, go off on many tangents, and impulsively make decisions. I also noticed many getting lost and constantly having to refer to their conference map about which room to go to for a particular session. In other words, there are a lot of people there who are just like you.

How Support Groups Can Help

There are several primary advantages of a good support group, including those described here.

1. **Members can understand.** Let's face it, most adults with ADD have "been there, done that," where most of the problems you face are concerned. They may have helpful ideas that never occurred to you before. Also, you may surprise yourself by having resolved issues that are still baffling to other members. With a collaborative spirit and good networking, a support group can be worth its weight in gold.

2. **Members may know about current research.** It can be difficult to be aware of the latest information on research that could be helpful to adults with ADD. But when you get a group of adults with ADD together, the probability greatly increases that at least one member knows about the latest research findings or even brings in copies to show everyone. Thus, a support group can be extremely helpful as a purveyor of important information. And if you can find a support group that has at least a few moms with ADD, then you have found yourself a gold mine of morale boosting.

3. **Members may recommend professionals.** Who is in a better position to know which psychiatrists, psychologists, and therapists are treating adult ADD than a group of adults who have been diagnosed with ADD? As a result, these individuals can swap advice and stories about the best and the worst of the helping professionals in your area.

One caveat: Do keep in mind that differences of opinion are natural; one person may dislike a therapist who she perceives as annoying, while another person may find that therapist very helpful. Whenever possible, don't rely on one person's opinion about a therapist.

Where to Find Support Groups

The best source for finding a support group in your area is CHADD. You can call them, or you can go to their website and look up the nearest support group to you. Here are some other ways to find support groups:

- Ask your physician if she knows of any support groups in the area.
- Check your local newspaper. Often local groups announce meeting times and places in a particular part of the newspaper, perhaps on a specific day like Wednesday or Friday. If you can't find such a section, call the newspaper and ask them if (and when) they do publish such information. And while you're at it, ask the newspaper staff if they know of any groups.

- Ask your clergyperson. Often members of the clergy know of many different self-help groups in the area. This is not always true but it doesn't hurt to ask!
- Ask your child's school, anonymously if you wish. Even if your child doesn't have ADD, the school counselor is probably aware of ADD groups in the area. Most ADD groups either work with adults with ADD or know about other groups who do.

Online Support Groups

Maybe there are no support groups in your area. But if you have access to the Internet, you may find enormous support from others with ADD who are out there in the online word and who may have the very information that you need. There are subsections of forums on America Online and an entire forum on CompuServe dedicated to children and adults with ADD.

In addition, there are "listservs" for people with ADD, including one specifically oriented to women with ADD. A *listserv* is a service that you "subscribe" to online (usually for no charge), and you will then receive all the electronic mail that anyone posts on that listserv. You can also post messages with questions and concerns and quickly receive feedback from other members.

To sign up for the ADDwomen listserv, go to <http://onelist.com/community/ addwomen>. This service also offers you the option of receiving daily digests of messages or reading messages on the bulletin board at your convenience. There is no cost.

Another listserv that may provide help is the AAADD-Focused list. To subscribe, go to <www.maillist.net/aadd.html>.

Until they joined an ADD support group, many people thought they were the "only ones" like themselves and were amazed that other people also lose items, forget things, and behave impulsively. ADD support groups provide not only moral support but also information that you might not find otherwise, whether it's about treatment, coping strategies, or something else.

In this chapter, I also described coaches, individuals who assist you on an individual basis to set goals and meet them. You may also find a professional organizer would be the right answer for you, a person who can show you where things should go and teach you how to keep things that way.

Appendix A
Recommended Books

The ADHD Parenting Handbook: Practical Advice for Parents, by Colleen Alexander-Roberts (Taylor Publishing, 1995). Plenty of useable, helpful hints for the non-ADD mother and the mother with ADD.

Charter Schools: Creating Hope and Opportunity for American Education, by Joe Nathan (Jossey-Bass Publishers, 1999). To learn more about charter schools, read this book.

The Complete Idiot's Guide to Organizing Your Life (2nd edition), by Georgene Lockwood (Alpha Books, 1999). If you thought organizing was boring, you haven't read this entertaining and helpful book.

If I Could Just Get Organized! Home Management Hope for Pilers and Filers, by Karen Jogerst (Rubies Publishing, P.O. Box 709, Manhattan, MT 59741; 1999). If you don't want to give up your piles, this upbeat book may help.

Understanding Girls with AD/HD, by Kathleen Nadeau, Ph.D., Ellen B. Littman, Ph.D., and Patricia O. Quinn, M.D. (Advantage Books, 1999). The book you need if your daughter has ADD.

Women with Attention Deficit Disorder: Embracing Disorganization at Home and in the Workplace, by Sari Solden (Underwood Books, 1995). This book pioneered acceptance that women can and do have attention deficit disorder.

You Mean I'm Not Lazy, Crazy or Stupid?!: A Self-Help Book for Adults with Attention Deficit Disorder, by Kate Kelly and Peggy Ramondo (New York: Scribner, 1995). An entertaining and helpful book written by women who truly understand.

Magazines and Journals

ADDvance: A Magazine for Women with Attention Deficit Disorder. Edited by Kathleen Nadeau, Ph.D. and Patricia Quinn, M.D. and published six times per year. A don't-miss publication for women with ADD, whether you're a mom or not.
   ADDvance: A Magazine for Women with ADD
   1001 Spring St., Suite 118
   Silver Spring, MD 20910
   Tel: (888) 238-8588
   Website: www.addvance.com

ADHD Research Update
An electronic newsletter published by a psychologist; summarizes research on children with attention deficit disorder.

Free samples available online at www.helpforadd.com/nresearch.htm.

Attention!
8181 Professional Place, Suite 201
Landover, MD 20785
Tel: (800) 233-4050
Official publication of CHADD (Children and Adults with Attention Deficit Disorder)

Journal of Attention Disorders
Multi-Health Systems, Inc.
908 Niagara Falls Blvd.
North Tonawanda, NY 14120-2060
An academic journal that offers the results of clinical studies.

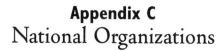

Appendix C
National Organizations

Children and Adults with Attention Deficit Disorder (CHADD)
8181 Professional Place, Suite 201
Landover, MD 20785
Tel: (800) 233-4050 or (301) 306-7070
Fax: (301) 306-7090
Website: www.chadd.org

National Alliance for the Mentally Ill (NAMI)
Colonial Place Three
2107 Wilson Blvd., 3rd Floor
Arlington, VA 22201
Tel: (703) 524-7600
Website: www.nami.org

Messies Anonymous
5025 SW 114th Ave.
Miami, FL 33316

Tel: (800) 637-7292
Fax: (305) 273-7671
Website: www.messies.com/

National Attention Deficit Disorder Association
1788 Second St., Ste. 200
Highland Park, IL 60035
Tel: (847) 432-2332
E-mail: mail@add.org
Website: www.add.org

National Association of State Directors of Special Education (NASDSE)
1800 Diagonal Rd., Suite 320
Alexandria, VA 22314
Tel: (703) 519-3800
Website: www.NASDE.org

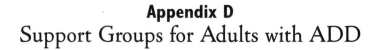

Appendix D
Support Groups for Adults with ADD

The following groups are not all specifically oriented to moms with ADD. In addition, a few groups encompass adults and children with ADD. Phone numbers are not included for all groups, because some leaders asked that their numbers not be listed.

Alabama
CHADD of Tri-County Alabama
Tel: (334) 867-3898

Alaska
Anchorage CHADD
Tel: (907) 338-1491

Arizona
Adults with ADD (Division of South Mountain CHADD)
(480) 753-5045

Mountain CHADD
(covers Phoenix, Tempe, Ahwatukee, and Chandler)
Parent Support Group contact: (480) 706-5162
E-mail: KFlessor1@aol.com

Arkansas
CHADD of Central Arkansas
Tel: (501) 835-9000

California
CHADD of Bakersfield
P.O. Box 10563
Bakersfield, CA 93389
Tel: (805) 328-0438

Support ADD/ADHD (in association with CHADD NorCal)
Tel: (925) 472-9444

Colorado
Support Group (Durango area)
Tel: (970) 259-7147
E-mail: deedee@outerbounds.net

Connecticut
CHADD of Greater Danbury
P.O. Box 4427
Danbury, CT 06811
E-mail: LoriLu725

District of Columbia
District of Columbia Chapter of Children and Adults with Attention Deficit Disorder (DC-CHADD)
Tel: (202) 319-9188
E-mail: Stephanye@weaveincorp.org
(Stephanye Snowden)

Florida
CHADD of Pinellas County

P.O. Box 8025
Seminole, FL 33775
Tel: (727) 789-7706

South Broward/North Dade CHADD
Tel: (954) 680-0799

Georgia
CHADD of Cherokee County
Tel: (770) 381-8687, ext. 08

CHADD of Cobb County
P.O. Box 670502
Marietta, GA 30062
Tel: (770) 381-8687, ext. 93

Illinois
Adult ADD Support Group
E-mail: DrJaksa@aol.com

Kansas
CHADD of Greater Kansas City
Tel: (913) 897-0917

CHADD of Wichita
Tel: (316) 722-3650

Kansas City Adult ADD Support Group
(Kansas City Metropolitan area)
Contact: Avner Stern, Ph.D. at (913)
345-1551
E-mail: godwin_bev@hotmail.com

Louisiana
ADDult (Baton Rouge area)
Tel: (225) 261-0613
E-mail: lacachadd@hotmail.com
Website: http://live.av.com/Clubs-
lacachadd

Maryland
CHADD of Baltimore County
Tel: (410) 377-0249

CHADD of Westminster/Owings Mills
740 David Ave.
Westminster, MD 21157
Tel: (410) 751-3820
Fax: (410) 840-0584

Massachusetts
Central Massachusetts CHADD
Tel: (508) 755-0688

Michigan
CHADD of Grand Rapids
Tel: (616) 248-2423

Minnesota
CHADD of the Twin Cities
Tel: (612) 922-5761

New Hampshire
Central New Hampshire CHADD
Tel: (603) 224-4153

Seacoast CHADD
Tel: (603) 430-8787

New York
Greater Rochester Attention Deficit
Disorder Association
Warmline: (716) 251-2322
Fax: (716) 352-2055
E-mail: megndick@juno.com

Ohio
Michael Romaniuk, Ph.D.
Group Facilitator, Adult ADD Support
Group
Akron General Medical Center
400 Wabash Ave.
Akron, OH 44307
Tel: (800) 221-4601, ext. 47602 OR
(330) 344-7602
E-mail: mromaniuk@agmc.org
Website: www.akrongeneral.org/add/

Oklahoma
CHADD of Green County
P.O. Box 877
Jenks, OK 74037
Tel: (918) 298-2423

Rhode Island
RI ADDults
Austin Donnelly, M.Ed.
Hotline: (401) 463-8778
E-mail: Adon@aol.com

Virginia
CHADD of Northern Virginia
P.O. Box 2645
Fairfax, VA 22031
Tel: (703) 641-5451

Washington
ADDult Support of Washington
P.O. Box 7804
Tacoma, WA 98407-7804
Tel: (253) 383-5332
E-mail: addult@addult.org
Website: www.addult.org

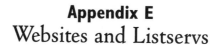

Websites and Listservs

A website is a place on the Internet devoted to a particular topic. A listserv is a list of people who voluntarily "subscribed" and receive by e-mail all messages sent by everyone on the listserv. It's impossible to list all possible websites that include information on ADD; so, I am offering only a sampling of what is available.

Websites

About.com: Attention Deficit Disorder
http://add.about.com/health/add/

ADD Coaching (Author/Coach Kate Kelly)
www.addcoaching.com/home.htm

ADDmirable Women
http://www.addmirablewomen.com/delphi.html

ADDvance: A Magazine for Women with Attention Deficit Disorder
www.addvance.com

Born to Explore: The Other Side of ADD
http://borntoexplore.org

Bouncing Brains
http://bouncingbrains.com

Canadian Professionals ADD Centre
www.usask.ca/psychiatry/CPADDC.html

Children and Adults with Attention Deficit-Hyperactivity Disorder (CHADD)
www.chadd.org

Global Assistive Devices (vibrating watch)
www.globalassistive.com/vb13.html

HADD-IT
(humorous site about ADD)
www.hadd-it.com/homepag.html

National Association of Professional Organizers
www.napo.net

National Association of State Directors of Special Education (NASDSE)
www.NASDSE.org

National Attention Deficit Disorder Association
www.add.org

Sari Solden's website
www.sarisolden.com

Taming the Triad (eduational site)
http://tamingthetriad.com

U.S. Charter Schools
www.uscharterschools.org/tech_assist/
menu_federal.htm

Listservs and Usenet Groups

ADDmirable Women

List guidelines/subscription info:
http://www.addmirablewomen.com/
faq.html

Addwomen
To sign up, go to http://onelist.com/
community/addwomen

AADD-FOCUSED mailing list (for
adults with ADD)
www.maillist.net/aadd.html

Appendix F
Summer Camps with Programs for Kids with ADD

The following camps report that they either specialize in or have programs for children with ADD. Listing in this book is not an endorsement of any camp, and parents should be sure to thoroughly check out each camp (listed here or found elsewhere) before signing up their child.

Camp Northwood
132 State Route 365
Remsen, NY 13438
Tel: (315) 831-3621
E-mail: gfeltwww.nwood.com
Website: www.nwood.com

Camp Nuhop
404 Hillcrest Drive
Ashland, OH 44805
Tel: (419) 289-2227
E-mail: info@campnuhop.org
Website: www.campnuhop.org

New Jersey YMHA-YWHA Camps
21 Plymouth St.
Fairfield, NJ 07004-1615
Tel: (973) 575-3333
E-mail: rlc@njycamps.org

SOAR
Director, LD and AD/HD Services
P.O. Box 388
Balsam, NC 28707-0388
Tel: (828) 456-3435
Fax: (828-456-3449
Website: www.soarnc.org

Summit Camp
110-45 71st Rd., Suite 1G
Forest Hills, NY 11375
Tel: (718) 268-0020 or (800) 323-9908
E-mail: summitcamp@aol.com
Website: www.castlepoint.com/summit/

Vail Valley Learning Camp
P.O. Box 1146
Vail, CO 81658
Tel: (970) 926-2706
E-mail: info@learningcamp.com
Website: www.learningcamp.com

Appendix G
State Contacts for Charter School Information

Alaska
Ms. Marjorie Menzi
Charter School Liaison
Alaska Dept. of Education
801 West 10th St.
Juneau, AK 99801-1894
Tel: (907) 465-8720

Arkansas
Dr. Gayle Potter
Associate Director, Curriculum &
Instruction
Arkansas Dept. of Education
#4 State Capitol Mall, Rm. 106A
Little Rock, AR 72201
Tel: (501) 682-4558
E-mail: gpotter@arkedu.k12.ar.us

California
Ting Sun
Charter Schools Office
California Dept. of Education
560 J St., Ste. 170
Sacramento, CA 95814
Tel: (916) 445-6761
E-mail: tsun@cde.ca.gov

Colorado
Mr. Bill Windler
Senior Consultant, School Improvement

Colorado Dept. of Education
201 E. Colfax Ave.
Denver, CO 80203
Tel: (303) 866-6631

Connecticut
Ms. Jennifer C. Niles
Charter School Program Manager
Division of School Improvement
Connecticut Dept. of Education
P.O. Box 2219
Hartford, CT 06145-2219
Tel: (860) 566-1233

District of Columbia
Nelson Smith
Executive Director
DC Public Charter School Board
1717 K St., NW, Ste 802
Washington, DC 20006
Tel: (202) 887-5011

Delaware
Dr. Larry Gabbert
Charter School Administrator
Delaware Dept. of Education
P.O. Box 1402
Dover, DE 19903
Tel: (303) 739-4629
E-mail: lgabbert@state.de.us

Florida
Mr. Tracey Bailey
Director, Office of Public School Choice
Florida Education Center
325 Gaines St., Rm. 522
Tallahassee, FL 32399
Tel: (850) 414-0780

Georgia
Beverly Schenger
Coordinator, Charter Schools Program
Georgia Dept. of Education
2054 Twin Towers East
Atlanta, GA 30334
Tel: (404) 656-4151
E-mail: charter.schools@doe.k12.ga.us

Hawaii
Mr. Art Kaneshiro
Director, School/Community-Based Management
Hawaii Dept. of Education
1270 Queen Emma St., #409
Honolulu, HI 96813
Tel: (808) 586-3124

Idaho
Carolyn Mauer
Idaho State Dept. of Education
P.O. Box 83720
Boise, ID 83720-0027
Tel: (208) 332-6974
E-mail: cmauer@sde.state.id.us

Illinois
Gail Lieberman
Senior Policy Advisor
Illinois State board of Education
100 North First St.
Springfield, IL 62777
Tel: (217) 782-5053

Kansas
DR. Phyllis Kelly
Charter School Coordinator
Kansas State Dept. of Education
120 Southeast 10th Ave.
Topeka, KS 66612-1182

Tel: (785) 296-3069
E-mail: pkelly@smtpgw.ksbe.state.ks.us

Louisiana
Kathy Matheny
Louisiana State Board of Elementary and
Secondary Education
P.O. Box 94064
Baton Rouge, LA 70804-9064
Tel: (505) 219-4540
E-mail: kmathene@mail.doe.state.la.us

Massachusetts
Mr. Scott Hamilton
Associate Commissioner for Charter
Schools
Massachusetts Dept. of Education
1 Ashburton Place, Rm. 1403
Boston, MA 02108
Tel: (617) 727-0075

Michigan
Ms. Joan May
Supervisor, Public School Academy
Program
Michigan State Dept. of Education
P.O. Box 30008
Lansing, MI 48909
Tel: (517) 373-4631

Minnesota
Traci Laferriere
Charter School Coordinator
Minnesota Dept. of Children, Families
and Learning
Highway 36 West
Roseville, MN 55113
Tel: (651) 582-8217

Missouri
Susan Cole
Coordinator of State Programs
Missouri State Dept. of Education
P.O. Box 480
Jefferson City, MO 65102
Tel: (573) 751-3175
E-mail: scole@mail.dese.state.mo.us

Mississippi
Richard Roberson
Charter School Consultant
Mississippi Dept. of Education
P.O. Box 771
Jackson, MS 39205
Tel: (601) 359-3501
E-mail: rroberson@mde.k12.ms.us

Nevada
Holly Walton Buchanan
Nevada Dept. of Education
700 E. 5th St.
Carson City, NV 89701-5096
Tel: (702) 687-9186

New Hampshire
Ms. Patricia Busselle
Administrator
New Hampshire Dept of Education
State Office Park South
101 Pleasant St.
Concord, NH 03301
Tel: (603) 271-3879

New Jersey
Cynthia Hoenes
Program Specialist
Office of Innovative Programs and
Practices
New Jersey State Dept. of Education
P.O. Box 500
Trenton, NJ 08625-0500
Tel: (609) 292-5850

New Mexico
Dr. Michael A. Kaplan
Director, Alternative Education Unit
New Mexico Department of Education
300 Don Gaspar
Santa Fe, NM 87501-2786
Tel: (505) 827-6576
E-mail: mkaplan@sde.sytate.nm.us

North Carolina
Dr. Grova L. Bridgers
Office of Charter Schools
Dept. of Public Instruction

301 N. Wilmington St.
Raleigh, NC 27601-2825
Tel: (919) 715-1730

New York
Office of Elementary, Middle, Secondary
and Continuing Education
New York State Education Dept.
Education Building Annex, Rm. 875
Albany, NY 12234
Tel: (518) 474-5915
E-mail: emscgen@mail.nysed.gov

Ohio
Mr. John Rothwell
Community Schools Commission
Ohio Dept. of Education
65 S. Front St.
Columbus, OH 43215
Tel: (6514) 466-2937

Oklahoma
Oklahoma State Dept. of Education
2500 North Lincoln Blvd.
Oklahoma City, OK 73105-4599
Fax: (405) 521-6205
E-mail: sandy garrett@mail.sde.state.ok.us

Oregon
Randy Hamisch
Oregon Dept. of Education
Public Service Building
255 Capitol St. NE
Salem, OR 97310
Tel: (503) 378-8004 ext. 222
E-mail: Randy.hamisch@state.or.us

Pennsylvania
Dr. Tim Daniels
Charter Schools Program
Pennsylvania Dept. of Education
333 Market St.
Harrisburg, PA 17126
Tel: (717) 783-9781

Rhode Island
Mr. Steve Nardelli
Charter School Administrator

Rhode Island Dept. of Education
255 Westminster St.
Providence, RI 02903
Tel: (401) 222-4600, ext. 2015

South Carolina
Catherine Samulski
Education Associate
State Dept. of Education
1429 Senate St., Rm. 605
Columbia, SC 29201
Tel: (803) 734-8277
E-mail: csamulski@sde.state.sc.us

Texas
Mr. Brooks Flemister
Senior Director for Charter Schools
Texas Education Agency
1701 N. Congress Ave.
Austin, TX 78701
Tel: (512) 463-9575
E-mail: bflemist@mail.tea.state.tx.us

Utah
Doug Bates
Associate Superintendent
Planning and Project Services Division
Utah State Office of Education
250 East 500 South
Salt Lake City, UT 84111
Tel: (801) 538-7762

Virginia
Dr. Yvonne Thayer
Policy and Public Affairs
Virginia Dept. of Education

P.O. Box 2120
Richmond, VA 23218-2120
Tel: (804) 786-5392
E-mail: ythayer@pen.k12.va.us

Wisconsin
Dennis G. Wicklund
Charter School Consultant
Dept. of Public Instruction
125 S. Webster St.
P.O. Box 7841
Madison, WI 53707-7841
Tel: (608) 266-5728

Wyoming
Kathy Scheurman
Charter School Supervisor
State Dept of Education
2300 Capitol Ave.
2nd Floor, Hathaway Bldg.
Cheyenne, WY 82002
Tel: (307) 777-7843

Puerto Rico
Ms. Nilda Baez De Morales
Executive Director
Educational Reform Institute
Puerto Rico Dept. of Education
P.O. Box 192379
San Juan, PR 00919
Tel: (787) 765-9772

Appendix H
Products That May Be Helpful

Natural Alarm Clocks (wake you up with increased light)
Bio-Brite, Inc.
4350 East-West Highway, Suite 401W
Bethesda, MD 20814
Tel: (800) 621-LITE

Special Watches
Vibralite Watches
Global Assistive Devices, Inc.
4950 North Dixie Highway, Suite 121
Fort Lauderdale, FL 33334-3947
Website: http://catalog.globalassistive.com

WatchMinder watch
P.O. Box 19565-226
Irvine, CA 92623-9565
Tel: (800) 961-0023
Website: www.watchminder.com

Bibliography

Alberts-Corush, Jody, Ph.D., et al. "Attention and Impulsivity Characteristics of the Biological and Adoptive Parents of Hyperactive and Normal Control Children." *American Journal of Orthopsychiatry* 56, no. 3 (July 1986): 413–423.

Alexander-Roberts, Colleen. *ADHD & Teens: A Parent's Guide to Making It through the Tough Years.* Dallas, TX: Taylor Publishing, 1995.

Ambert, Anne-Marie, Ph.D. *The Effect of Children on Parents.* New York: The Haworth Press, 1992.

Arnold, L. Eugene. "Sex Differences in ADHD: Conference Summary." *Journal of Abnormal Child Psychology* 24, no. 5 (October 1996): 555–569.

Baumgaertel, Anna, M.D. "Alternative and Controversial Treatments for Attention-Deficit/Hyperactivity Disorder." *Pediatric Clinics of North America* 46, no. 5 (October 1999): 977–992.

Bellak, Leopold, ed. *Psychiatric Aspects of Minimal Brain Dysfunction in Adults.* New York: Grune & Stratton, 1979.

Biederman, Joseph, M.D., et al. "Familial Association between Attention Deficit Disorder and Anxiety Disorders" *American Journal of Psychiatry* 2 (February 1991): 251–256.

Bloomingdale, Lewis M., and James M. Swanson *Attention Deficit Disorder: Current Concepts and Emerging Trends in Attentional and Behavioral Disorders of Childhood.* New York: Pergamon Press.

Braswell, Lauren, and Michael L. Bloomquist. *Cognitive-Behavioral Therapy with ADHD Children: Child, Family and School Interventions.* New York: The Guilford Press, 1991.

Buntman, Peter H., MSW, ACSW. *Living with ADHD Children: A Handbook for Parents.* (Los Alamitos, CA: Center for Family Life, Inc., 198).

Conners, C. Keith, Ph.D., and Juliet L. Jett. *Attention Deficit Hyperactivity Disorder. In Adults and Children: The Latest Assessment and Treatment Strategies.* Kansas City, MO: Compact Chemicals, 1999.

Cramond, Bonnie. "Attention-Deficit Hyperactivity Disorder and Creativity—What Is the Connection?" *Journal of Creative Behavior* 28, no. 3 (Third Quarter 1994): 193–210.

Eisenberg, Ronni. *The Overwhelmed Person's Guide to Time Management.* New York: Penguin Books, 1997.

Erk, Robert R. "Attention Deficit Hyperactivity Disorder: Counselors, Laws, and Implications for Practice." *Professional School Counseling* 2, no. 4 (April 1, 1999): 318–338.

Faraone, Stephen V., Ph.D., et al. "A Family-Genetic Study of Girls with DSM-III Attention Deficit Disorder." *American Journal of Psychiatry* 148, no. 1 (January 1991): 112–117.

Faraone, Stephen V., Ph.D., et al. "Toward Guidelines for Pedigree Selection in Genetic Studies of Attention Deficit Hyperactivity Disorder." *Genetic Epidemiology* 18, no. 1 (2000): 1–16.

Fisher, Barbara C., and Ross A. Beckley. *Attention Deficit Disorder: Practical Coping Methods.* Boca Raton, FL: CRC Press, 1999.

Hallowell, Edward M., M.D., and John J. Ratey, M.D. *Driven to Distraction.* New York: Pantheon Books, 1994.

Harris, Judith Rich. *The Nurture Assumption: Why Children Turn Out the Way They Do.* New York: Touchstone, 1998.

Hartmann, Thom. *Healing ADD: Simple Exercises That Will Change Your Daily Life.* Grass Valley, CA: Underwood Books, 1998.

Hechtman, Lily, M.D., F.R.C.P.C., ed. *Do They Grow Out of It? Long-Term Outcomes of Childhood Disorders.* Washington, DC: American Psychiatric Press, 1996.

Hoagwood, Kimberly, et al. "Treatment Services for Children with ADHD: A National Perspective." *Journal of the American Academy of Child and Adolescent Psychiatry* 39, no. 2 (February 2000).

Horacek, H. Joseph Jr. *Brainstorms: Understanding and Treating the Emotional Storms of Attention Deficit Hyperactivity Disorder from Childhood through Adulthood.* Northvale, N: Jason Aronson Inc, 1998.

Ingersoll, Barbara D., Ph.D. *Daredevils and Daydreamers: New Perspectives on Attention-Deficit/Hyperactivity Disorder.* New York: Doubleday, 1998.

Jackson, Belinda, and David Farrugia. "Diagnosis and Treatment of Adults with Attention Deficit Hyperactivity Disorder." *Journal of Counseling and Development* 75 (March/April 1997): 312–319.

Katherine, Anne. *Boundaries: Where You End and I Begin.* New York: Fireside/Parkside, 1991.

Kelly, Kate, and Peggy Ramundo. *The ADDed Dimension: Everyday Advice for Adults with ADD.* New York: Scribner, 1997.

Kelly, Kate, and Peggy Ramundo. *You Mean I'm Not Lazy, Stupid Or Crazy?!: A Self-Help Book for Adults with Attention Deficit Disorder.* New York: Scribner, 1995.

Kendall, Judy. "Sibling Accounts of Attention Deficit Hyperactivity Disorder (ADHD)." *Family Process* 38 (Spring 1999): 117–136.

Kern, Roy M., et al. "Lifestyle, Personality, and Attention Deficit Hyperactivity Disorder in Young Adults." *Journal of Individual Psychology* 55, no. 2 (Summer 1999): 186–199.

"Kids' ADHD Care Gets a Wake-Up Call." *Science News,* 156, no. 25 & 26 (December 18 and 25, 1999), 388.

Khouzam, Hani R. "Attention Deficit Hyperactivity Disorder in Adults: Guidelines for Evaluation and Treatment." *Consultant* 37, no. 8, (August 1997): 2159–2165.

Levine, Merle Langbord, B.A., M.Ed. "The Effect of the ADHD Child on the Mother" Unpublished paper presented at the 1993 CHADD conference in San Diego, CA.

Levitan, Robert D., et al. "Seasonal Affective Symptoms in Adults with Residual Attention-Deficit Hyperactivity Disorder." *Comprehensive Psychiatry* 40, no. 4 (July 1, 1999): 261–267.

Lockwood, Georgene. *The Complete Idiot's Guide to Organizing Your Life.* New York: Alpha Books, 1999.

Maté, Gabor, M.D. *Scattered: How Attention Deficit Disorder Originates and What You Can Do about It.* New York: Dutton, 1999.

Nadeau, Kathleen G., Ph.D., ed. *A Comprehensive Guide to Attention Deficit Disorder in Adults: Research, Diagnosis, and Treatment.* New York: Brunner/Mazel Publishers, 1995.

Nadeau, Kathleen G., Ph.D. *ADD in the Workplace: Choices, Changes and Challenges.* New York: Brunner/Mazel Publishers, 1997.

Nadeau, Kathleen G., Ph.D., et al. *Understanding Girls with Attention Deficit Hyperactivity Disorder.* Silver Spring, MD: Advantage Books, 1999.

Nathan, Joe. *Charter Schools: Creating Hope and Opportunity for American Education.* New York: Jossey-Bass Publishers, 1999.

Neuman, Rosalind J. "Evaluation of ADHD Typology in Three Contrasting Samples: A Latent Class Approach." *Journal of the American Academy of Child and Adolescent Psychiatry* 38, no. 1 (January 1999): 25–34.

Pfiffner, Linda J., et al. "Association of Parental Psychopathology to the Comorbid Disorders of Boys with Attention Deficit-Hyperactivity Disorder." *Journal of Consulting Psychology* 67, no. 6 (December 1999): 881–893.

Roberts, M. Susan, Ph.D., and Gerard H. Jansen, Ph.D. *Living with ADD: A Workbook for Adults with Attention Deficit Disorder.* Oakland, CA: New Harbinger Publications, 1997.

Seidman, Larry J. "Neuropsychological Function in Adults with Attention-Deficit Hyperactivity Disorder." *Biological Psychiatry* 44 (1998): 260–268.

Sharp, Wendy S., et al. "ADHD in Girls: Clinical Comparability of a Research Sample." *Journal of the American Academy of Child and Adolescent Psychiatry* 38, no. 1 (January 1999): 40–47.

Solden, Sari, M.S., M.F.C.C., *Women with Attention Deficit Disorder: Embracing Disorganization at Home and in the Workplace.* Grass Valley, CA: Underwood Books, 1995.

Sudderth, David B., M.D. and Joseph Kandel, M.D. *Adult ADD: The Complete Handbook.* Rocklin, CA: Prima Publishing, 1997.

Swanson, J.M., et al. "Attention-Deficit Hyperactivity Disorder and Hyperkinetic Disorder." *The Lancet* 351 (February 7, 1998): 429–433.

Swedo, Susan M.D., and Henrietta Leonard, M.D. *It's Not All In Your Head: Now Women Can Discover the Real Causes of Their Most Commonly Misdiagnosed Health Problems.* San Francisco: HarperSanFrancisco, 1996.

Taylor, John F., Ph.D. *Helping Your Hyperactive /Attention Deficit Child.* Rocklin, CA: Prima Publishing, 1994.

Thapar, Anita, et al. "Genetic Basis of Attention Deficit and Hyperactivity." *British Journal of Psychiatry,* 174 (February 1999): 105–111.

Thomas, J. Lawrence, and Christine Adamec. *Do You Have Attention Deficit Disorder?* New York: Dell, 1996.

Thornton, James. *Chore Wars: How Households Can SHARE the Work & Keep the Peace.* Berkeley, CA: Conari Press, 1997.

U.S. Department of Justice. "Enforcing the ADA: A Status Report from the Department of Justice." July–September 1999.

Vitanza, Stephanie A., Ph.D., and Charles A. Guarnaccia. "A Model of Psychological Distress for Mothers of Children with Attention-Deficit Hyperactivity Disorder." *Journal of Child and Family Studies* 8, no. 1 (1999): 27–46.

Von Oech, Roger. *A Kick in the Seat of the Pants: Using Your Explorer, Artist, Judge & Warrior to Be More Creative.* New York: Harper & Row, Publishers, 1986.

Walker, Craig, Ph.D. "Genetics and Gender in ADHD: Genetics Matter; Gender Doesn't." Unpublished paper presented at the 1999 annual ADDA meeting.

Weiss, Dr. Lynn. *Attention Deficit Disorder in Adults: Practical Help for Sufferers and Their Spouses.* Dallas, TX: Taylor Publishing, 1992.

Weiss, Gabrielle, and Lily Trokenberg Hechtman. *Hyperactive Children Grown Up: ADHD in Children, Adolescents, and Adults.* New York: The Guilford Press, 1993.

Weiss, Margaret, M.D., Ph.D., et al. *ADHD in Adulthood: A Guide to Current Theory, Diagnosis and Treatment.* Baltimore, MD: Johns Hopkins University Press, 1999.

Wender, Paul H., M.D. *Attention-Deficit Hyperactivity Disorder in Adults.* New York: Oxford University Press, 1995.

Wilens, Timothy E., M.D. *Straight Talk about Psychiatric Medications for Kids.* New York: Guilford Press, 1999.

Wolraich, Marl L., M.D., et al. "Comparison of Diagnostic Criteria for Attention-Deficit Hyperactivity Disorder in a County-Wide Sample." *Journal of the American Academy of Child & Adolescent Psychiatry* 35, no. 3 (1996): 319–324.

Young, Susan. "Psychological Therapy for Adults with Attention Deficit Hyperactivity Disorder." *Counselling Psychology Quarterly* 12, no. 2 (1999): 183–190.

Index

ADA (Americans with Disabilities Act)(1990), 75, 76, 136, 137, 140
ADD
 adopted children and, 104
 diagnosing, 6, 16–18, 80–81, 173–174
 difficult or painful emotions that may accompany, coping with, 145–157
 fears of, 154–155
 friendliness of job toward, 72–74
 getting outside help with, 167–174
 good aspects of, 19–29
 living with, 15–16
 moms with. *See* Mom(s), with ADD
 problems with
  primary, determining, 59–60
  solutions to
   ADD coaches and, 188
   family and, 58, 64–65
   high-tech, 54–55
   low-tech, 53–54
   organizational, 31–39. *See also* Organization
   professional organizers and, 187
   support groups and, 188–190. *See also* Support groups
  without solutions, 106
 society's acceptance of
  girls or women and, 3–4
  men or boys and, 3, 15
  time for, 6–7
 surprises about, 27
 symptoms of, listing, 181–183
 terminology regarding, 17
 thought of as myth, 5–7
 treatment of

  biofeedback and, 186
  children and, 80–81
  dietary changes and, 185–186
  homeopathy and, 186
  medication and. *See* Medication(s)
  professional help and. *See* Medical doctor(s); Psychiatrist(s); Psychologist(s); Social worker; Therapist
 women with. *See also* Mom(s), with ADD
 screening checklist for, 17–18
ADD coaches, 188
ADD in the Workplace: Choices, Changes, and Challenges (Nadeau), 51
Adderall, 178
ADHD Gender Study Project, 7
Adolescent(s), 115–122
 acting as, bad behavior versus, 115–118
 behavior by, 115–118
  sexual, 122
 boundaries for, 118–119
 changing needs of, adapting to, 119–120
 curfew and, 121
 dating and, 121
 disciplining, 120–122
 expectations and, 118–119
 manipulation by, 116
 offering choices to, 117–118, 120–122
 open-door policy and, 118–119
 personal property and, 119
 privacy and, 118–119
 schoolwork and, 122
 things that upset, 117
Adopted children, ADD and, 104
Aggression, reports of not listened to, 90–91
Alternative medicines, 184–185

America Online, ADD forums on, 190
American Psychiatric Association, 16
Americans with Disabilities Act (ADA)(1990), 75, 76, 136, 137, 140
Anger
    child's misbehavior and, 146–147
    coping with, 146–147
    management of, 9, 109, 146–147
Antidepressant medications, 178
Appointment boards, 53
Attention deficit disorder. See ADD
Attention-deficit hyperactivity disorders, 16–17. See also ADD

Baby(ies)/toddler(s). See also Children
    catching in act of accidentally being good, 98–99
    with mom who has ADD, 93–102
    potty training and, 95
    setting limits for, 96–100. See also Discipline
Baumgaertel, Anna, 185
Behavior
    adolescent, 115–118, 122
    of children. See Children, behavior of
    sexual, 122
Biederman, Joseph, 85
Biofeedback, 186
Birthdays, children's, 160
Bluntness, 13
Blurting out, 50–51
Boundaries
    for adolescent, 118–119
    personal, 66–67
        violating, 66–67
        remembering, 66–67
"Brainstorms," 109
Bykofsky, Sheree, 43

Caffeine, paradoxical reactions to, 94
Calendars, 53
    multiple, 46–47
CHADD (Children and Adults with Attention Deficit Disorder), 170, 172, 188–190
Chaos
    crisis of, creating plan to deal with, 153–154
    making rules versus, 63
Charity, donating old toys to, 84
Charter school(s)
    defined, 130–131
    learning more about, 135
    origin of, 134
    parental awareness of, 134–135
    pros and cons of, 133–134
    state laws regarding, 131–133

Charter Schools Expansion Act (1998), 131
Charts, 5
    discipline and, 100
Checklist
    ADD symptoms and, 183
    for listening, 48–49
    screening for women with ADD and, 17–18
Childcare
    choosing, 70
    facility providing
        bad, 71–72
        discipline at, 71, 100
        evaluating, 70–72
        location of, 70
        finding, 69–72
        picking up child from, 72
Children. See also Baby(ies)/toddler(s)
    with ADD
        diagnosis of, 80–81
        getting to take medication. See Medication(s)
        helping with organization, 84
        with mom who has ADD too, 79–85
        with other problems on top of, 84–85
        school accommodations for, 128, 136–141. See also School(s); Teacher(s)
            asking for, stigma and, 138
        siblings of, 85
            key issues with, 89–92
            too much responsibility given to, 90
        treatment of, 80–81
    adopted, ADD and, 104
    behavior of
        ADD-like, exhibited by non-ADD child, 88
        bad
            mom blamed for, 5
            your temper and, 146–147
        common childhood ploys and, 109–112
        effects of, on parents, 107–112
        parental control over, 9
        parents' reaction to, 107–112
        which mirrors that of mom with ADD, 105–106
    birthdays and, 160
    care for, while at work. See Childcare
    commitment to, deep, 28
    disciplining. See Discipline
    embarrassment and, 105
    holidays and, 159–160
    medication and. See Medication(s)
    non-ADD, with mom who has ADD. See Non-ADD child whose mom has ADD
    parties and, 160
    school-age, parenting of, 103–113. See also Parenting
    sickness and, 162–163

summer vacations and, 160–161
traveling with, 161–162
when they don't like you, 104
when you don't like, 104
Children and Adults with Attention Deficit Disorder (CHADD), 170, 172, 188–190
Chore Wars: How Households Can Share the Work and Keep the Peace (Thornton), 58
Cleaning, child does most or all of, 87–88
Clinton, Bill, 131, 136, 139
Clipboards, 53–54
Clothes, spicy, 51–52
Clutter
coping with, 13
disposal of, benefit of, 39
volume of, 35–39
Communication, rules for, 111–112
Compassion, 24–25
The Complete Idiot's Guide to Organizing Your Life (Lockwood), 32
Comprehensive Psychiatry, 148
Compuserve, ADD forum on, 190
Computer organizers, 54–55
Concentration, ignoring outside distractions and, 9
Cooking, child does most or all of, 87–88
Corporal punishment, 99–100
Cramond, Bonnie, 23
Creativity
boosters of, 24
as feature of people with ADD, 22–24
smashers of, 24
society's appreciation and, 23–24
solving problems using, 43, 58
Crying, 150
Curfew, 121
Curiosity, 22, 43
Cylert (pemoline), 178

Dating, adolescent, 121
Daytimers, 53
Decision-making
about weekends, by non-ADD child, 88
collaberating in, 49–50
impulsivity and, 11–12
Desipramine, 178
Desoxyn (methampethamine), 178
Dexedrine (dextroamphetamine), 177–178
DextroStat, 178
Diagnostic and Statistical Manual of Mental Disorders: DSM-IV (American Psychiatric Association), 16–17, 20
Dietary changes, 185–186
Dietary Supplement Health and Education Act (1994), 184

Digital voice recorders, 55
Diplomacy, 10
Discipline, 13
of adolescent, 120–122
catching child in act of accidentally being good and, 98–99
charts and, 5, 100
at childcare facility, 71, 100
choices in, offering, 96
forms of, 96–100
point systems and, 5, 100
self-, 8
of small children, 96–100
difficulty in, 96
spanking and, 99–100
time-outs and, 96–98
withholding privileges and, 99
Distractions, ignoring, 9, 14
Do You Have Attention Deficit Disorder? (Thomas), 25
Documentation, for effective communication, 49
Donahue, Phil, 8
Douglas, Ann, 70, 72
Drug abuse, prevention of, 177
DSM-IV (Diagnostic and Statistical Manual of Mental Disorders: DSM-IV)(American Psychiatric Association), 16–17, 20

Edison, Thomas, 24
Education. *See* School(s); Teacher(s)
Education for All Handicapped Children Act (1975), 136
Embarrassment, 105
Empathy, 24–25
The Encyclopedia of Child Abuse, 156
Energy, high, 27–28

Family, 57–67. *See also* Home
history of, shared humorous events from, 27
issues for, 65
meeting of, 64–65
members of, working out solutions with, 64–65
problem-solving in, 58
responsibilities in, stress and, 152–153
thinking about work, while with, 74–75
Family and Medical Leave Act (1993), 75
Family Process, 89–91, 156
Faraone, Stephen, 85
Fault, dealing with, 111
FDA (Food and Drug Administration), 176, 184
"Feingold diet," 185

Files
  categories of, 34
  vanishing piles into, 32–33
Firm, being, 63
500 Terrific Ideas for Organizing Everything
  (Bykofsky), 43
Focusing, 14
Food and Drug Administration (FDA), 176,
  184
Forgetting, 11. *See also* Remembering
Frustration, feelings of incompetence and, 147–
  152

General Accounting Office, charter school
  information and, 135
Genetic Epidemiology, 85
Giving in, 63
Goals, writing down, 60–61
Grocery shopping, 107
Guidance counselor, letter to, 138–140
Guilt
  moms and, 5
  saying no and, 42–43
  self-blame and, 147

Hairspray (movie), 97
Harris, Judith Rich, 108
Holidays, coping with, 159–160
Home. *See also* Family
  creative problem-solving at, 58
  responsibilities in, stress and, 152–153
  schooling your child in, 135
  skills to work on at, 61–63
  thinking about work, while at, 74–75
Home schooling, 135
Homeopathy, 186
Horacek, H. Joseph, 109
Humor, sense of, 25–26
Hyperactivity, 14–15
Hyperfocusing, 20–21
Hyperreactivity
  adaptations to, 52
  to stimuli, 51–52

IDEA (Individuals with Disabilities Education
  Act), 136, 137, 138, 140
IEP (Individual Education Plan), 136, 141
*If I Could Just Get Organized! Home Manage-
  ment Hope for Pilers & Filers* (Jogerst), 33

Impulsivity, 24
  decision-making and, 11–12

saying yes and, 43
Incompetence, feelings of, frustration and,
  147–152
Individual Education Plan (IEP), 136,
  141
Individuals with Disabilities Education Act
  (IDEA), 136, 137, 138, 140
IRS Publication No. 552, 33

Job(s), 69–76
  ADD-friendliness of, 72–74
  childcare and. *See* Childcare
  environment of, good, 72–73
  laws that affect workers and, 75–76
  problems with, 73–74
  responsibilities of, stress and, 152–153
  thinking about, while at home, 74–75
Jogerst, Karen, 33
Journal of Creative Behavior, 23
*Journal of the American Academy of Child and
  Adolescent Psychiatry*, 83

Kelly, Kate, 66, 124, 188
Kendall, Judy, 89–91, 156
Keys, losing, 40–41

Learned helplessness, 147, 148
Leshner, Alan I., 177
Levine, Merle Langbord, 79–80
Listening
  checklist for, 48–50
  hearing what others mean to say and,
    150
  lashing out versus, 150–152
  learning and, 47–50
Listserv, 190
Living in the now, 28
Lockwood, Georgene, 32
Losing items, 12
  child's ploy regarding, 110
  keys and, 40–41
  reasons for, 39–42
  retracing steps and, 39–40

Manipulation, good, bad manipulation versus,
  116
Mate, Gabor, 45
Matlen, Terry, 21
Medical doctor(s). *See also* Psychiatrist(s)
  degree earned by, 171
  doctor's attitude regarding, 171

failure of, to diagnose ADD, 173–174
finding, 169–170, 174
meeting with, 170–171
screening, 169–170
Medication(s), 175–186. *See also Individual
  medications*
  alternative, 184–185
  antidepressant, 178
  benefits possible from, 176
  child's getting for mom, 87
  combinations of, 179
  effectiveness of, evaluating, 181–183
  giving to child, 81–83
    fear of, 82
    in morning, tip for giving, 105
    thinking you're bad for, 82–83
  how doctors select, 179
  pros and cons of, 180–181
  psychiatrists and, 169
  self-administered by child, 87
  side effects of, 181
  substance abuse prevention and, 177
  taking
    fear of, 176–177
    on time, 180–181
Memory
  forgetting and, 11. *See also* Remembering
  tricks to aid, 32–33
Merle Levine Academy, Inc., 79
Messiness, coping with, 13
Mistakes, 105
Mittens, 106
Mom(s)
  with ADD
    adolescents and. *See* Adolescent(s)
    with baby(ies)/toddler(s), 93–102. *See also*
      Baby(ies)/toddler(s)
      expectations of, 101–102
    with children who don't have ADD, 86–92.
      See also Non-ADD child whose mom has
      ADD
    with children who have ADD too, 79–85,
      89–92. *See also* Children with ADD
      medication for child and. *See* Medica-
        tion(s)
      over-identifying with, 81–82
    difficulties in being, 4–5
    disciplining child and. *See* Discipline
    embarrassment and, 105
    fault and, 111
    fears of ADD and, 154–155
    getting outside help and, 167–174
    good mothers versus bad mothers and,
      154–157
    grocery shopping and, 107, 111
    high energy and, 27–28

hyperactivity and, 14–15
inability of, to solve problem, 106
inward view of, 66–67
magic wish related to ADD and, 14
meanness and, 111
mistakes made by, 105
myths and realities about, 29
number of, 7
parenting by. *See* Parenting
realities and myths about, 29
self-doubts and, 100
surprises about ADD and, 27
teachers' understanding of, 127–128. *See
  also* School(s); Teacher(s)
time disconnect and, 44
typical, traits and characteristics of, 10–16,
  19–29
under-identifying with non-ADD child and,
  86
wishes of, 14
bad, traits of, 155–157
diplomacy and, 10
good
  good mom's mother versus, 10
  traits of, 7–10, 157
guilt and, 5
listening by, 47–50. *See also* Listening
neatness and, 9–10
problems blamed on, 4
reliability and, 8
self-control and, 9
self-discipline and, 8
tact and, 10
world's expectations from, 7–10
Monuteaux, Michael, 85
Mother. *See* Mom(s)
Multiple calendars, 46–47
Multitasking ability, 29

Nadeau, Kathleen G., 26, 46, 51, 87, 130, 153–
  154, 160
NAMI (National Alliance for the Mentally Ill),
  170, 172
Napoleon, 43
National Alliance for the Mentally Ill (NAMI),
  170, 172
National Institute of Mental Health, 177
National Institute on Drug Abuse (NIDA),
  177
"Natural medicines," 184–185
Neatness, 9–10
Negative self-talk, 153
NIDA (National Institute on Drug Abuse),
  177

Non-ADD child whose mom has ADD, 86–92
  ADD-like behavior exhibited by, 88
  all or most decisions about weekend made by,
    88
  classic problems with, 88–89
  with feeling that life is chaotic and will never
    improve, 91–92
  invisible, 90
  low profile maintained by, 88
  most or all of cooking and cleaning done by,
    87–88
  need of, for mom, 88
  "parentalizing" by, 86–88
  parenting of, challenges of, 86–89
  trying to be perfect and, 89
Notes
  taking, 49
  to yourself, writing, 74
*The Nurture Assumption: Why Children Turn
  Out the Way They Do* (Harris), 108

Open-door policy, 118–119
Organization
  clutter versus, 35–39
  donating old toys to charity and, 84
  filing and. *See* Files
  helping child with ADD with, 84
  mail and, 34
  problems with
    particularly difficult, 106–107
    solutions to, 31–39
      creativity and, 43, 58
      high-tech, 54–55
      low-tech, 53–54
      professional organizers and, 187
  remembering and, 41–42
  of school-related items, 124–125

Pagers, 54
Palm Pilot, 54–55, 75
Parenting
  communication and, 111–112
  complications in, 5
  of non-ADD child whose mom has ADD, 86–89
  realities of, 103–106
  rules and, 112–113. *See also* Rule(s)
  school and. *See* School(s); Teacher(s)
  of school-age child, 103–113
Patience, working on, 62
Pediatric Clinics of North America, 185
Personal property, adolescent and, 119
Piles
  giving up, 33–35
  vanishing of, into files, 32–33

Plan creation, 59–61
  to deal with crisis of chaos, 153–154
Planners, 53
Point systems, discipline and, 5, 100
Positive people, 148
Potty training, 95
Privacy, adolescents and, 118–119
Privileges, withholding, 99
Procrastination, 12
Professional help. *See* Medical doctor(s);
    Psychiatrist(s); Psychologist(s); Social worker;
    Therapist
Professional organizers, 187
Project(s)
  critique of, 37–38
  doing in parts, 37
Property, personal, adolescent and, 119
Prozac (fluoxetine), 178
Psychiatrist(s)
  failure of, to diagnose ADD, 173–174
  finding, 169–170, 174
  function of, 168–169
  meeting with, 170–171
  screening, 169–170
Psychologist(s)
  capabilities of, 172–173
  degree earned by, 171, 172
  failure of, to diagnose ADD, 173–174
  screening, 172–173

Questions
  to ask doctor, 170–171
  asking, for clarification, 49

Rage, 146. *See also* Anger
Rash, 181
Recorders, voice, digital, 55
Rehabilitation Act (1973), Section 504 of, 136–
    137, 138
Reliability, 8
Remembering
  boundaries and, 66–67
  difficulty with, 11
  organizing and, 41–42
  reminders and, 74–75
  tricks to assist in, 32–33
Reminders, setting up, 74–75
Rewards for yourself, 38
Ritalin (methylphenidate), 85, 89, 177
  studies on children taking, 83
Rule(s)
  for communication, 111–112
  creating and sticking with, 112–113
  curfew, 121

for family meeting, 65
making, chaos versus, 63
posting, 113
self-test on, 112–113
writing down, 113

SAD (seasonal affective disorder), 148
Saying no
fear of, 42–43
guilt and, 42–43
saying yes versus, 42–44. *See also* Saying yes
Saying yes
high frequency of, 42–45
impulsively, 43
saying no versus, 42–44. *See also* Saying no
Scattered: How Attention Deficit Disorder Originates and What You Can Do About It (Mate),
45
Schedule(s)
multiple calendars and, 46–47
time and, 45–47. *See also* Time
unchangeables and, 47
School(s). *See also* Teacher(s)
adolescent and, 122
charter. *See* Charter school(s)
child's adjustment to, 123–125
guidance counselor in, letter to, 138–140
home schooling and, 135
homework and, 122, 124, 125, 128–130,
139–140
problems at, 125–126
requirements for children with ADD and, 128,
136–141
failure of school to comply with, 140–
141
summer vacations from, 160–161
superintendent of, letter to, 140–141
unreasonable demands from, 126
when they don't work, 130–135
Science projects, 128–130. *See also* Homework
Seasonal affective disorder (SAD), 148
Section 504 of Rehabilitation Act of 1973, 136–
137, 138
Selective serotonin reuptake inhibitors (SSRIs),
178
Self-blame, guilt and, 147
Self-control, 9
Self-discipline, 8
Self-doubts, 100
Self-talk, negative, 153
Sensitivity, 24–25
Sexual behavior, 122
Sick children, 162–163
Skills to work on at home, 61–63
Sleep, getting enough, 149–150

SOAR, 161
Social worker
degree earned by, 171, 173
service provided by, 173
Society
acceptance by
of ADD, 6–7
boys and men and, 3, 15
girls and women and, 3–4
appreciation of, for creative people, 23–24
expectations of, from mothers, 7–10
how moms and guilt are seen by, 5
Solden, Sari, 3, 24–25, 66–67
screening checklist of, for women with ADD,
17–18
Spanking, 99–100
Spicy clothes, 51–52
Spontaneity, 24. *See also* Impulsivity
Spontaneity deficit disorder, 26
SSRIs (selective serotonin reuptake inhibitors),
178
Strategies, workable, developing, 61
Stress, 152–154
exorcising with exercise, 152
work and family responsibilities and, 152–
153
Substance abuse, prevention of, 177
Summer camp, 161
Superintendent of schools, letter to, 140–
141
Support groups, 188–190
finding, 189–190
how they can help, 189
online, 190
Systems
creating, 61
overload of, 153

Tact, 10
Taskier, Claudia, 84
Teacher(s). *See also* School(s)
accusatory, 126
conferences with parents and, 126–128
neat-aholic, 126
problems with, 125–126
schoolwork form for use with, 139–140
unreasonable demands from, 126
Teenager. *See* Adolescent(s)
Temper. *See also* Anger
child's misbehavior and, 146–147
maintaining, 9
Therapist
degree earned by, 171, 173
service provided by, 173

Therapy, 85
    considering, self-test for, 167–168
    sources of, 168–173. *See also* Medical
        doctor(s); Psychologist(s)
Thomas, James Lawrence, 25
Thomas, Marlo, 8
Thoreau, Henry David, 46
Thornton, James, 58
Time
    curfew, 121
    flexibility and, 45–47
    losing track of, 11
    managing, 45–47
    for medication, 180–181
    moms with ADD and, 44
    multiple calendars and, 46–47
    to pick up child from childcare, 72
    as a problem, 46–47
    timers and, 45
    watches and, 55
Time-outs, 96–98
Timers, 45
Toys, old, donating to charity, 84
Trash barrels, 38
Travel with children, 161–162
Tricyclics, 178

United States Department of Education
    charter schools and

    information about, 135
    studies about, 133
    handicapped children and, 136, 137
    modifications for children with ADD and,
        128
United States Department of Justice
    "Enforcing the ADA" report of,
        75
    toll-free line of, for information about
        ADA, 76
The Unofficial Guide to Childcare (Douglas),
    70

Voice recorders, digital, 55

Walker, Craig W., 7
Watches, 55
Wellbutrin (buproprion), 85,
    178
White-noise generators, 55
Women with Attention Deficit Disorder (Solden),
    3, 25
Work. *See* Job(s)

Yellow stickies, 40
You Mean I'm Not Lazy, Stupid, or Crazy?!
    (Kelly), 188